Handbook of
SUPPORTIVE CARE
in PEDIATRIC
ONCOLOGY

Editor-in-Chief
OUSSAMA ABLA, MD
Assistant Professor of Paediatrics, University of Toronto
Staff Oncologist, Division of Haematology/Oncology
Department of Paediatrics, The Hospital for Sick Children
Toronto, Ontario

Associate Editors
VICKY BREAKEY, MD, FRCP(C)
Fellow, Division of Haematology/Oncology
Department of Paediatrics, The Hospital for Sick Children
Toronto, Ontario

L. LEE DUPUIS, PRH, MSCPHM, FCSHP
Clinical Pharmacist, Division of Haematology/Oncology
Department of Pharmacy, The Hospital for Sick Children
Toronto, Ontario

AHMED NAQVI, MBBS, DCH, MCPS, MRCP, FRCPCH
Assistant Professor of Paediatrics, University of Toronto
Staff Oncologist, Division of Haematology/Oncology
The Hospital for Sick Children
Toronto, Ontario

TONY H. TRUONG, MD, MPH, FRCP(C)
Clinical Fellow, Division of Haematology/Oncology
Department of Paediatrics, The Hospital for Sick Children
Toronto, Ontario

JONES AND BARTLETT PUBLISHERS
Sudbury, Massachusetts
BOSTON   TORONTO   LONDON   SINGAPORE

World Headquarters

Jones and Bartlett
  Publishers
40 Tall Pine Drive
Sudbury, MA 01776
978-443-5000
info@jbpub.com
www.jbpub.com

Jones and Bartlett
  Publishers Canada
6339 Ormindale Way
Mississauga, Ontario
L5V 1J2
Canada

Jones and Bartlett
  Publishers International
Barb House, Barb Mews
London W6 7PA
United Kingdom

Jones and Bartlett's books and products are available through most bookstores and online book-sellers. To contact Jones and Bartlett Publishers directly, call 800-832-0034, fax 978-443-8000, or visit our website www.jbpub.com.

Substantial discounts on bulk quantities of Jones and Bartlett's publications are available to corporations, professional associations, and other qualified organizations. For details and specific discount information, contact the special sales department at Jones and Bartlett via the above contact information or send an email to specialsales@jbpub.com.

Copyright © 2010 **SickKids**® The Hospital for Sick Children

All rights reserved. No part of the material protected by this copyright may be reproduced or uti-lized in any form, electronic or mechanical, including photocopying, recording, or by any infor-mation storage and retrieval system, without written permission from the copyright owner.

The authors, editor, and publisher have made every effort to provide accurate information. How-ever, they are not responsible for errors, omissions, or for any outcomes related to the use of the contents of this book and take no responsibility for the use of the products and procedures de-scribed. Treatments and side effects described in this book may not be applicable to all people; likewise, some people may require a dose or experience a side effect that is not described herein. Drugs and medical devices are discussed that may have limited availability controlled by the Food and Drug Administration (FDA) for use only in a research study or clinical trial. Research, clini-cal practice, and government regulations often change the accepted standard in this field. When consideration is being given to use of any drug in the clinical setting, the healthcare provider or reader is responsible for determining FDA status of the drug, reading the package insert, and re-viewing prescribing information for the most up-to-date recommendations on dose, precautions, and contraindications, and determining the appropriate usage for the product. This is especially important in the case of drugs that are new or seldom used.

This book is a general guide only and should never be a substitute for the skill, knowledge, and experience of a qualified medical professional dealing with the facts, circumstances, and symp-toms of a particular case.

Production Credits
Executive Publisher: Christopher Davis
Sr. Editorial Assistant: Jessica Acox
Production Editor: Daniel Stone
Sr. Marketing Manager: Barb Bartoszek
V.P., Manufacturing and Inventory Control:
  Therese Connell

Composition: DBS
Printing and Binding: Malloy, Inc.
Cover Printing: Malloy, Inc.

Cover Credits
Cover Design: Scott Moden
Cover images: © Anna Jurkovska/ShutterStock, Inc.

Library of Congress Cataloging-in-Publication Data
Abla, Oussama.
  HSK handbook of supportive care in pediatric cancer / Oussama Abla.
      p. ; cm.
  Includes bibliographical references and index.
  ISBN-13: 978-0-7637-5985-8
  ISBN-10: 0-7637-5985-6
  1. Cancer in children—Handbooks, manuals, etc. 2.
Cancer—Complications—Handbooks, manuals, etc. 3.
Cancer—Treatment—Handbooks, manuals, etc. I. Title. II. Title: Handbook
of supportive care in pediatric cancer.
  [DNLM: 1. Child—Handbooks. 2. Neoplasms—complications—Handbooks. 3.
Neoplasms—therapy—Handbooks. QZ 39 A152h 2010]
  RC281.C4A25 2010
  618.92'994—dc22
                                              2009022815
  6048

Printed in the United States of America
13 12 11 10 09   10 9 8 7 6 5 4 3 2 1

Contents

Contributors

Oussama Abla, MD
Assistant Professor of Paediatrics
University of Toronto
Staff Oncologist
Division of Haematology/Oncology
Department of Paediatrics
The Hospital for Sick Children
Toronto, Ontario

Reshma Amin, MD, FRCP(C)
Paediatric Respirology Fellow
Master's of Clinical Epidemiology Student
Department of Paediatric Respiratory Medicine
The Hospital for Sick Children
University of Toronto
Toronto, Ontario

Rand Askalan, PhD, MD, FRCP(C)
Staff Neurologist
Children's Stroke Program
Clinician-Scientist Investigator
The Hospital for Sick Children
Toronto, Ontario

Ute Bartels, MD
Assistant Professor of Paediatrics
University of Toronto
Staff Physician
Brain Tumor Program
Division of Haematology/Oncology
Department of Paediatrics
The Hospital for Sick Children
Toronto, Ontario

Leonardo R. Brandao, MD
Assistant Professor of Paediatrics
University of Toronto
Thrombosis, Division of Haematology/Oncology
Department of Paediatrics
The Hospital for Sick Children
Toronto, Ontario

Vicky R. Breakey, MD, FRCP(C)
Fellow
Division of Haematology/Oncology
Department of Paediatrics
The Hospital for Sick Children
Toronto, Ontario

Michaela Cada, MD, FRCP(C), FAAP, MPH
Co-Chief Fellow
Division of Haematology/Oncology
Department of Paediatrics
The Hospital for Sick Children
Toronto, Ontario

Manuel D. Carcao, MD, FRCP(C), MSc
Associate Professor of Paediatrics (Haematology/Oncology)
University of Toronto
Associate Director
Haemophilia Clinic
Associate Scientist
Research Institute
The Hospital for Sick Children
Toronto, Ontario

Amy Lee Chong, LRCP & SI, MB, BCh, BAO(NUI), MRCPI(PAEDS)
Fellow
Division of Haematology/Oncology
Department of Paediatrics
The Hospital for Sick Children
Toronto, Ontario

Debbie Chong, BSc, BScPhm, RPh, ACPR
Pharmacist Haematology/Oncology and Bone Marrow Transplant
The Hospital for Sick Children
Toronto, Ontario

Claire De Souza, BSc, MD, FRCP(C)
Assistant Professor
University of Toronto
Staff Psychiatrist
Department of Psychiatry
The Hospital for Sick Children
Toronto, Ontario

L. Lee Dupuis, PRh, MScPhm, ACPR, FCSHP
Associate Professor
Leslie Dan Faculty of Pharmacy
University of Toronto
Clinical Pharmacy Specialist
Department of Pharmacy
Division of Haematology/Oncology
Project Investigator
Child Health Evaluative Sciences, Research Institute
The Hospital for Sick Children
Toronto, Ontario

Fraser Golding, MD, FRCP(C)
Assistant Professor of Paediatrics
University of Toronto
Staff Cardiologist
The Hospital for Sick Children
Toronto, Ontario

Ronald Grant, MD, FRCP(C)
Staff Oncologist
Head, Solid Tumor
Division of Haematology/Oncology
Department of Paediatrics
The Hospital for Sick Children
Toronto, Ontario

Hartmut Grasemann, MD, PhD
Associate Professor of Paediatrics
University of Toronto
Staff Physician
Paediatric Respiratory Medicine
The Hospital for Sick Children
Toronto, Ontario

Gloria J. Green, MSc, RD
Clinical Dietitian
Haematology/Oncology Programme
The Hospital for Sick Children
Toronto, Ontario

Sumit Gupta, MD, FRCP(C)
Fellow
Division of Haematology/Oncology
Department of Paediatrics
The Hospital for Sick Children
Toronto, Ontario

Valerie Langlois, MD, FRCP(C)
Assistant Professor of Paediatrics
University of Toronto
Staff Physician
Division of Nephrology
Department of Paediatrics
The Hospital for Sick Children
Toronto, Ontario

Wendy Lau, MBBS, FRCP(C)
Assistant Professor
University of Toronto
Director
Transfusion Medicine
Department of Paediatric Laboratory Medicine
The Hospital for Sick Children
Toronto, Ontario

Simon C. Ling, MBChB
Assistant Professor of Paediatrics
University of Toronto
Staff Gastroenterologist
Division of Gastroenterology, Hepatology & Nutrition
The Hospital for Sick Children
Toronto, Ontario

Basem Naser, MBBS, FRCP(C)
Assistant Professor
University of Toronto
Director of Acute Pain Service and Staff Anesthesiologist
Department of Anesthesia and Pain Medicine
The Hospital for Sick Children
Toronto, Ontario

Ahmed Naqvi, MBBS, DCH, MCPS, MRCP, FRCPCH
Assistant Professor of Paediatrics
University of Toronto
Staff Oncologist
Division of Haematology/Oncology
The Hospital for Sick Children
Toronto, Ontario

Dragos Predescu, MD
Cardiology Fellow
Division of Cardiology
Department of Paediatrics
The Hospital for Sick Children
Toronto, Ontario

Angela Punnett, MD, FRCP(C)
Assistant Professor of Paediatrics
University of Toronto
Staff Physician
Division of Haematology/Oncology
Department of Paediatrics
The Hospital for Sick Children
Toronto, Ontario

Lillian Sung MD, PhD, FRCP(C)
Associate Professor of Paediatrics
Division of Haematology/Oncology
University of Toronto
Scientist, Program in Child Health Sciences, Hospital for Sick
    Children
Department of Paediatrics
The Hospital for Sick Children
Toronto, Ontario

Tracey Taylor, BScPhm, ACPR, RPh
Staff Pharmacist
Division of Haematology/Oncology and Bone Marrow Transplant
    Clinics
The Hospital for Sick Children
Toronto, Ontario

Tony H. Truong, MD, MPH, FRCP(C)
Clinical Fellow
Division of Haematology/Oncology
Department of Paediatrics
The Hospital for Sick Children
Toronto, Ontario

Stacey L. Urbach, MD, MPH, FRCP(C)
Assistant Professor of Paediatrics
University of Toronto
Staff Physician
Division of Endocrinology
The Hospital for Sick Children
Toronto, Ontario

Jocelyne Volpe, RN, BScN, MN
Clinical Nurse Specialist/Nurse Practitioner
Division of Haematology/Oncology
Department of Paediatrics
The Hospital for Sick Children
Toronto, Ontario

Sheila Weitzman, MB, BCh, FCP(SA), FRCP(C)
Professor of Paediatrics
University of Toronto
Associate Director Clinical Affairs for the Division of
    Haematology/Oncology
The Hospital for Sick Children
Toronto, Canada

Suzan Williams, MD, MSc, FRCP(C)
Assistant Professor of Paediatrics
University of Toronto
Thrombosis, Division of Haematology/Oncology
Department of Paediatrics
The Hospital for Sick Children
Toronto, Ontario

Elyse Zelunka, BSc, Phm, RPh
Pharmacist
Division of Haematology/Oncology
    and Bone Marrow Transplant Clinics
The Hospital for Sick Children
Toronto, Ontario

Preface

This handbook provides a practical approach to the clinical management of the problems unique to childhood cancer. It will be an essential resource to pediatric residents, fellows, and nurse practitioners especially while they are on call, at night. It deals specifically with acute complications of pediatric cancer and its therapy. The main objective is to have a quick reference for the management of oncologic and hematologic emergencies, and for symptom management in children with cancer.

This handbook, hopefully, will serve as a comprehensive approach and knowledge base for all physicians, trainees, nurse practitioners, and nurses who care for children with cancer on a daily basis.

Oussama Abla, MD

c h a p t e r   1

Acute Allergic Reactions

Oussama Abla and Ahmed Naqvi

Outline

- Common Etiologies in Pediatric Cancer Patients
- Precautions
- Clinical Presentation
- Initial Management
- Follow-Up

Common Etiologies in Pediatric Cancer Patients

- Chemotherapeutic agents: L-asparaginase (*E. coli*, *Erwinia*, PEG), etoposide (VP16), bleomycin, carboplatin, vinorelbine.
- Monoclonal antibodies: rituximab, alemtuzumab (Campath), gemtuzumab (Mylotarg).
- Antithymocyte globulin (ATG), gamma globulin (IV IG).
- Antibiotics: penicillins, cephalosporins, vancomycin.

- Blood products: packed red blood cells, platelets, granulocyte transfusions, fresh-frozen plasma, cryoprecipitates, fibrinogen, and coagulation factor concentrates (factor VIII, factor IX).

Precautions

Prior to the administration of drugs and products that increase the risk of allergic reactions:

- Assess the patients for previous allergic reactions.
- Have readily available the following:
  - ○ Ambu bag.
  - ○ Suction apparatus.
  - ○ Oxygen supply.
  - ○ A good Intravenous access with running normal saline at a minimal rate to keep vein open.
  - ○ IV injectable diphenhydramine, hydrocortisone, and epinephrine (1:1000), meperidine, ranitidine.
  - ○ Acetaminophen oral liquids and tablets.
  - ○ IV Normal saline vials and bags.
- Calculate and document the doses of the above mentioned medicines. Have this information available in front of the patient's medical record.

When administering drugs such as ATG, alemtuzumab, gemtuzumab, or rituximab Premedications (diphenhydramine/hydrocortisone/acetaminophen) should be given 30 minutes prior to infusion.

Clinical Presentation

- Local reactions: urticaria, flushing, general pruritus, nasal congestion.

- Systemic reactions: chest tightness, cough, wheezing, tachypnea, hoarseness, stridor, laryngeal edema, fever, chills, nausea, vomiting, abdominal pain, tachycardia, cyanosis, and anxiety.
- Life-threatening anaphylaxis: upper respiratory obstruction, respiratory arrest, hypotension, arrhythmias, cardiac arrest.

Initial Management

- Urticaria and pruritus: Stop the infusion immediately and administer diphenyhdramine (1–2 mg/kg IV; maximum 50 mg/dose, 300 mg/day).
- Chills and fever: Slow the infusion temporarily and administer acetaminophen (10–15 mg/kg/dose PO every 4–6 h as needed) with meperidine (1 mg/kg IV every 4 h as needed).
- Consider adding ranitidine (1–2 mg/kg IV every 6–8 h) for severe reactions and inhaled salbutamol for bronchospasm.
- For anaphylaxis:
  ○ Stop the infusion immediately.
  ○ Monitor vital signs closely.
  ○ Secure airway and give oxygen; have intubation supplies ready, and intubate if clinically indicated.
  ○ Epinephrine 1:1000 (0.1 mg/kg), 0.01 ml/kg up to 0.5 ml intramuscularly (IM) into the thigh (more rapid absorption than the arm); IM route is better than subcutaneous. Repeat epinephrine within 5 min if there is no improvement or if the child's condition deteriorates.

- Hydrocortisone 5–10 mg/kg IV, and diphenhydramine 1–2 mg/kg IV (may repeat every 4–6 h as needed).
- For hypotension: give IV normal saline bolus 20 ml/kg, and keep patient in recumbent position with feet elevated. If persistently hypotensive after 60 ml/kg total of normal saline, consult critical care team and initiate dopamine infusion 2–10 mcg/kg/min.
- For life-threatening shock: administer intravenous epinephrine 1:10,000 at a dose of 0.01 mg/kg (0.1 ml/kg). IV epinephrine should only be given with cardiac monitoring and by a critical care specialist.

Follow-Up

- For mild reactions: observe the patient for 6–8 h; for severe reactions, observe for at least 24 h.
- Patients who react to *E. coli* L-asparaginase should be switched to PEG-asparaginase, and those who react to PEG should be switched to *Erwinia* and observed for 24–48 h. Hold asparaginase completely for persistent allergy to the drug.
- In case of severe allergy to ATG, alemtuzumab, gemtuzumeb or rituximab:
  - Hold the medication on that day, rechallenge the following day using adequate premedication under strict medical supervision.
- For some medicines e.g. etoposide or vancomycin, administering the drug at a slower rate (infusion over 2 hours) should be tried.
- Document the reaction in the patient's medical chart, and advise the patient to obtain medical alert identification if appropriate.

References

Chowdhury BA. Intramuscular versus subcutaneous injection of epinephrine in the treatment of anaphylaxis. *J Allergy Clin Immunol.* 2002;109(4): 720.

Hughes G, Fitzharris P. Managing acute anaphylaxis: new guidelines emphasize importance of intramuscular adrenaline. *BMJ.* 1999;319:1–2.

Sampson HA, et al. Summary report. In: Symposium on the Definition and Management of Anaphylaxis. *J Allergy Clin Immunol.* 2005;115:584–591.

Winbery SL, Lieberman PL. Histamine and antihistamines in anaphylaxis. *Clin Allergy Immunol.* 2002;17:287–317.

c h a p t e r 2

All-Trans Retinoic Acid (ATRA) Toxicity

Oussama Abla and Sheila Weitzman

Outline

- Introduction
- Retinoic Acid Syndrome
- Pseudotumor Cerebri (PTC)
- Uncommon Toxicities

Introduction

- Acute promyelocytic leukemia (APL) is a subtype of acute myeloid leukemia that is most commonly characterized by a fusion protein PML/RARα, resulting from the fusion of the PML gene on chromosome 15 with the retinoic acid receptor gene on chromosome 17. The fusion protein resulting from the translocation binds to downstream targets inhibiting differentiation of hematopoietic cells. Occasionally variant translocations exist, most also involving the RARα gene.

- Binding of all-trans retinoic acid (ATRA) to the fusion complex induces differentiation in the APL blasts with up to 90% complete remission rates. Addition of ATRA to chemotherapy, or more recently to arsenic, has revolutionized therapy of APL in those in whom the leukemic blasts contain translocations involving RARα. Those patients in whom the APL blasts lack such a translocation, or have a "blocking" translocation, require regular AML therapy possibly including stem cell transplantation.

- Differentiation of APL blasts in response to ATRA results in an increase in the absolute neutrophil count, which needs to be differentiated from that caused by acute infection.

ATRA is generally well tolerated except for two major toxicities:

- Retinoic acid syndrome (RAS).
- Increased intracranial pressure (pseudotumor cerebri).

Retinoic Acid Syndrome (RAS)

Clinical Presentation

- Major toxicity of ATRA; also called differentiation syndrome.
- Incidence: ranges from 6% to 26%, and tends to be higher in patients treated with ATRA alone (26%)

versus those treated with ATRA plus chemotherapy (6–15%).

- Defined as the presentation of any three of the following symptoms in the setting of ATRA administration:
  - Fever.
  - Weight gain.
  - Respiratory distress.
  - Interstitial pulmonary infiltrates.
  - Pleural and pericardial effusions.
  - Episodic hypotension.
  - Acute renal failure.
- Other manifestations:
  - Dry skin, pruritus, cheilitis.
  - Bone pain, arthralgias.
  - Elevated liver enzymes, cholesterol, and triglycerides.
  - Hypercalcemia.
- RAS occurs usually during induction therapy, from day 2 to day 35 (median, 7 days); it is rare during maintenance therapy.
- More common among patients who present with a high WBC, or develop rapid leukocytosis.
- It has been associated with an increased risk of extramedullary relapse, especially in the CNS. However, the latter risk may be due to improved survival from APL rather than directly to ATRA.
- RAS can lead to death from progressive hypoxemia and multiorgan failure if not promptly recognized and treated.
- In recent studies the mortality rate has been reduced to 5% owing to earlier recognition and prompt administration of dexamethasone.

Pathophysiology

Still poorly understood, but proposed mechanisms include the following:

- Cytokine secretion: Some clinical manifestations of ATRA syndrome (such as fever, hypotension, and effusions) suggest a role for interleukin-1β (IL-1β), IL-6, IL-8, and TNF-α release by APL cells undergoing differentiation with ATRA.
- Leukocyte emigration from blood: Depends on a cascade of interactions:
  - ATRA induces the expression of β_2-integrins (LFA-1, ICAM-2) on the leukocytes, resulting in adhesion to the endothelium.
  - ATRA up-regulates CD11b, CD18, and CD54 in APL cell lines causing increased adhesion to pulmonary endothelium. In fact, the pathologic findings of RAS resemble transfusion-related lung injury.
- Cathepsin G: A serine protease known to enhance capillary permeability; is stimulated in patients treated with ATRA.
- Monocyte chemotactic protein-1 (MCP-1): Secreted from alveolar epithelial cells, it is involved in the chemotactic transmigration of ATRA-treated cells toward alveolar cells.

Evaluation

- RAS should be considered in any patient who develops respiratory distress while on ATRA.
- Chest X-ray may show pulmonary edema/infiltrates or pleural or pericardial effusion.

- RAS is often difficult to diagnose: rule out pneumonia, sepsis, fluid overload, congestive heart failure, and acute respiratory distress syndrome.

Prevention

- In uncontrolled studies, a very low mortality rate due to RAS has been reported with the administration of prophylactic steroids to patients with an initial WBC $> 5 \times 10^9/l$, or in those patients who develop leukocytosis (WBC $> 10 \times 10^9/l$).
- Given the potential toxicity of prolonged steroid administration and the lack of prospective data, however, prophylaxis cannot be routinely recommended for all patients.

Treatment

At the earliest manifestations of RAS and prior to development of a full-blown syndrome, the following measures should be immediately undertaken:

1. Temporary discontinuation of ATRA.
2. Prompt initiation of dexamethasone (0.25 mg/kg/dose IV q 12 h for patients < 40 kg, or 10 mg IV q 12 h for ≥ 40 kg) for a minimum of 3 days or until resolution of symptoms.
3. Furosemide (0.5–1 mg/kg) when clinically indicated.
4. Whenever ATRA toxicity has resolved, restart the drug at 75 % of the initial dose. Recurrent episodes of RAS will result in holding ATRA again and restarting dexamethasone until toxicity resolves again. ATRA will then be resumed at 50 % of initial dose.

Challenges in Children

- Compliance: Some young patients cannot reliably swallow ATRA capsules:
  - Consult with local pharmacist.
  - Soften capsules.
  - Use G-tube as a last resort.
- Neurotoxicity: Pseudotumor cerebri, more frequent than in adults.

Pseudotumor Cerebri (PTC)

- Syndrome of increased intracranial pressure includes severe headaches, vomiting, blurred vision, and papilledema. The major risk is loss of vision, which may be irreversible if PTC is prolonged.
- Reported in 9% of pediatric patients, especially those younger than 10 years.
- Usually a diagnosis of exclusion: patient awake and alert; lack of focal neurologic signs except VI cranial nerve (abducens) palsy.
- Documented elevation of CSF pressure (> 200 mm of H_2O), with normal CSF composition.
- Normal CT head and no other identifiable causes of intracranial hypertension.

Management

- Obtain neurologic and ophthalmologic consultations immediately. Follow very carefully the visual field status of the patient.

- Consider brain MRI; rule out sagittal sinus thrombosis.
- Hold ATRA until PTC improves to grade 0 or 1 (mild headache).
- Start dexamethasone (see section on RAS for doses).
- Start acetazolamide or furosemide.
- Repetitive lumbar punctures with removal of CSF.
- If visual acuity deteriorates, consider lumboperitoneal shunt or optic nerve sheath fenestration.

Uncommon Toxicities

- Sweet's syndrome:
  - Characterized by fever, neutrophilia, painful erythematous cutaneous plaques, and dense dermal infiltrates of mature neutrophils.
  - Can involve the skin, muscles, lungs, kidneys, and fascia.
  - Can be associated with RAS.
  - Responds rapidly to steroid therapy.
- Thrombosis:
  - Splenic infarction, deep vein thrombosis, and pulmonary emboli have been reported with ATRA. Sinus venous thrombosis and cerebral infarction have also been reported sporadically; very important to rule it out in cases of suspicious PTC.
- ATRA-induced myositis.
- Osteonecrosis of the femoral head.
- Scrotal ulcers.
- Hemophagocytic syndrome (HLH) reported in adults treated with ATRA, in association with RAS.
- Paralytic ileus.

References

Astudillo L, Loche F, Reynish W, et al. Sweet's syndrome associated with retinoic acid syndrome in a patient with promyelocytic leukemia. *Ann Hematol.* 2002;81(2):111–114.

De Botton S, Dombret H, Sanz M, et al. Incidence, clinical features, and outcome of all-trans retinoic acid syndrome in 413 cases of newly diagnosed acute promyelocytic leukemia: the European APL Group. *Blood.* 1998;92:2712–2718.

Garcia-Suarez J, Banas H, Krsnik I, et al. Hemophagocytic syndrome associated with retinoic acid syndrome in acute promyelocytic leukemia. *Am J Hematol.* 2004;76:172–175.

Goldschmidt N, Gural A, Ben Yehuda D. Extensive splenic infarction, deep vein thrombosis and pulmonary emboli complicating induction therapy with all-trans retinoic acid (ATRA) for acute promyelocytic leukemia. *Leuk Lymphoma.* 2003;44(8):1433–1437.

Kannan K, Khan HA, Jain R, et al. All-trans retinoic acid induced myositis. *Br J Haematol.* 2005;131:560.

Parmar S, Tallman MS. Acute promyelocytic leukemia: a review. *Expert Opin Pharmacother.* 2003;4(8):1379–1392.

Sakakura M, Nishii K, Usui E, et al. Bilateral osteonecrosis of the head of the femur during treatment with retinoic acid in a young patient with acute promyelocytic leukemia. *Int J Hematol.* 2006;83(3):252–253.

Shimizu D, Nomura K, Matsuyama R, et al. Scrotal ulcers arising during treatment with all-trans retinoic acid for acute promyelocytic leukemia. *Int Med.* 2005;44(5):480–483.

Tallman MS, Andersen JW, Schiffer CA, et al. Clinical description of 44 patients with acute promyelocytic leukemia who developed the retinoic acid syndrome. *Blood.* 2000;95(1):90–95.

Tsai WH, Shih CH, Lin CC, et al. Monocyte chemotactic protein-1 in the migration of differentiated leukaemic cells toward alveolar epithelial cells. *Eur Respir J.* 2008;31(5):957–962.

Cardiac Complications

Dragos Predescu and Fraser Golding

Outline

- Bradycardia
- Tachycardia
- Shock
- Pericardial Effusion
- Congestive Heart Failure

Bradycardia

- Synonym: Low heart rate (HR).
- Definition: Heart rate lower than the 5th percentile for age (see Table 3-1).

Table 3-1   Normal heart rates in infants and children.

Age	Heart Rate Awake	Mean	Heart Rate Asleep
0–3 months	85–205	140	80–160
3 months to 2 years	100–190	130	75–160
2–10 years	60–140	80	60–90
> 10 years	60–100	75	50–90

Source: Courtesy of Chameides L, Hazinski MF, eds. *Pediatric Advanced Life Support.* Dallas American Heart Association, 1997.

Etiology

- Sinus bradycardia: Hypothermia, hypothyroidism, athletic heart.
- Medication: Antiemetics (e.g., ondansetron, others; see Table 3-2).
- Increased intracranial pressure (associated with hypertension).
- During recovery period after serious illnesses.
- Long QT interval with secondary 2:1 AVB:
  o Electrolyte imbalance.
  o Medication.
- Leukemic/lymphomatous infiltration of the conduction tissue.

Assessment

- Assess airway, breathing, and circulation:
  o Consider state of the child (e.g., awake, sleep, active, upset) and appropriateness of heart rate and responses to change in state.

Text continued on page 24

Table 3-2 Cardiac side effects of cancer drugs.

Drug	Cardiac Side Effect	EKG	Investigations/ Monitoring	Comments
Anthracyclines				
Doxo > Dauno	Acute/subacute injury: transient arrhythmia, pericarditis-myocarditis, acute LV failure. Chronic cardiotoxicity: dose-dependent cardiomyopathy. Late-onset ventricular dysfunction, arrhythmia, and sudden death	Sinus tachycardia, atrial and ventricular ectopy, atrial tachyarrhythmia, low QRS voltage, T wave flattening, QT prolongation, Afl, AF	Serial EKG and ECHO (SF, EF, VCFc), cardiac enzymes and biomarkers	Torsade: late after treatment, women, hypokalemia, concomitant treatment with azoles
Epirubicine	CHF			Less cardiotoxicity compared with doxo/dauno
Idarubicin	CHF, arrhythmias, angina, acute myocardial infarction (AMI)			Same as above. Asymptomatic decrease in LVEF

(continued)

Table 3-2 (continued).

Drug	Cardiac Side Effect	EKG	Investigations/ Monitoring	Comments
Anthracyclines (continued)				
Mitoxantrone	Arrhythmias, CHF, AMI, EKG changes	Sinus tachycardia non-specific ST-T wave changes		Low-amplitude, high-frequency signals in the terminal portion of the QRS complex and ST segment
Alkylating agents				
Cyclophos-phamide	Tachycardia, CHF, chest pain, pericarditis, hemorrhagic cardiac necrosis	Sinus tachy, small voltage QRS, ST segment elevation, nonspecific ST-T wave changes	Increased cardiac enzymes (50%)	No report of late cardiotoxicity
Ifosfamide	CHF, SVT, pulseless tachycardia, pleural effusion	SVT, possible VT, decreased QRS voltage	Fluid intake, daily weighing, serum creatinine, electrolytes, EKG	CHF heralded by raise in creatinine levels. Discontinuation of Ifos reversed the cardiac abnormalities and these did not recur.

Cisplatin	Palpitations, chest pain, dyspnea, hypotension, arrhythmia, AMI	Intraventricular block, ST-T wave changes, T wave inversion	EKG, cardiac enzymes (CK-MB), electrolytes (Mg)	May happen at any time from hours after the first infusion is complete to up to 18 months after the completion of a cycle. Events do not seem to be dose related.
Mitomycin	CHF		Serial ECHO	Prior doxo therapy. Occurs weeks after multiple doses of mitomycin
Carmustine	Chest pain (myocardial ischemia), hypotension, sinus tachycardia	EKG changes suggestive for ischemia	BP, EKG, cardiac enzymes	Cardiotoxicity should be considered, especially when used in high doses in bone marrow transplant preparatory regimens.
Busulfan	CHF, palpitations, cardiac tamponade, pulmonary congestion, cardiomegaly, pericardial effusion, constrictive pericarditis, endocardial fibrosis	Peaked P waves and flat T waves (chronic)	Serial ECHO	

(continued)

Table 3-2 (continued).

Drug	Cardiac Side Effect	EKG	Investigations/ Monitoring	Comments
Alkylating agents (continued)				
Chlorme-thine	Persistent tachycardia, junctional or atrial ectopy	Supraventricular ectopy	Same as for anthracy-clines	
Antimetabolites				
Fluorouracil	Myocardial ischemia (angina, AMI, hypotension, cardiogenic shock), atrial and ventricular arrhythmias	Ischemic changes, sinus tachycardia, decreased QRS amplitude, QT prolongation, atrial fibrilation, ventricular arrhythmias. They return to normal after discontinuation of administration.	EKG, cardiac enzymes	More common after high doses in continuous infusion than after bolus doses. Majority of patients have angina during administration. Symptoms resolve after discontinuation of infusion but recur in 90% of cases when infusion restarted. May be more severe than previously.

Cytarabine	Pericardial effusion, CHF, pleural effusion, arrhythmia, acute respiratory distress	EKG changes suggestive for pericarditis	Serial ECHO, EKG, cardiac enzymes in symptomatic patients	Cardiotoxicity with high doses
Antimicrotubule agents				
Paclitaxel	Arrhythmias, dysautonomia, AMI, RBBB, LBBB	Sinus bradycardia, AVB, SVT, atrial flutter, AF, VT, VF, LBBB, RBBB	EKG monitoring, cardiac enzymes in symptomatic patients	Cardiotoxicity unrelated with dose. Bradycardia mostly asymptomatic. Paclitaxel doesn't exhibit a cumulative dose effect. Increases doxo toxicity.
Etoposide	Hypotension, AMI	Changes consistent with ischemia	BP during and immediately after the infusion; cardiac enzymes in symptomatic patients	Increase infusion time, IV fluids, discontinuation of infusion
Teniposide	Hypotension, arrhythmia		BP during and immediately after the infusion; EKG	Increase infusion time, IV fluids, discontinuation of infusion
Vinca alkaloids	AMI, pulmonary edema, arrhythmia, autonomic cardioneuropathy	EKG changes suggestive for ischemia, AF	EKG monitoring, cardiac enzymes in symptomatic patients	Cardiotoxicity is not dose related. AMI only with continuous infusions of vindesine.

(continued)

Table 3-2 (continued).

Drug	Cardiac Side Effect	EKG	Investigations/ Monitoring	Comments
Others				
Amsacrine	Atrial and ventricular arrhythmias, CHF, bradycardia, hypotension, cardiac arrest	QT prolongation, nonspecific ST-T changes, VT, AF, VF	EKG; serial ECHO if symptoms of CHF; serum potassium	Hypokalemia may increase risk of arrhythmia
Cladribine	CHF		Serial ECHO if symptoms of CHF	
Asparaginase	AMI (rare)	EKG changes suggestive for ischemia	EKG monitoring, cardiac enzymes in symptomatic patients	
Tretinoin	Arrhythmia, hypotension, hypertension, CHF, myocarditis, pulmonary hypertension. Retinoic acid syndrome (fever, respiratory distress, weight gain, peripheral edema, pleural-pericardial effusions, AMI)	Arrhythmia, EKG changes suggestive for pericarditis/ischemia	Monitor leucocytosis, DIC	

Pentostatin	Angina/AMI, CHF, arrhythmias, fluid overload	AF, atrial flutter, extrasystole	Monitor I/O; EKG monitoring, cardiac enzymes in symptomatic patients	Increased cardiotoxicity in association with cyclophosphamide
Trastuzumab	CHF, palpitations, tachycardia		No standard guidelines: clinical, EKG, serial ECHO	
Docetaxel	CHF, AF	AF	EKG monitoring	Toxicity increased when associated with anthracyclines. No autonomic dysfunction
Thalidomide	Pulmonary hypertension			
Tyrosine kinases inhibitors	LV dysfunction up to CHF		Serial ECHO	Reversible
Gemcitabine	AF, pericardial effusion, noncardiogenic pulmonary edema	AF, PR, ST-T changes	Serial EKG. Monitoring of symptoms	In adults, after infusion. Antiarrhythmic therapy was required for AF.
Arsenic trioxide	QT interval prolongation, torsade de pointes, CHB	QT interval prolongation, torsade de pointes, CHB	Baseline EKG. Monitor QT interval	

- A simple test to assess cardiovascular reactivity is have the child stand for 2 minutes and assess heart rate and blood pressure before and after. The heart rate should increase and blood pressure should not decrease more than 10 mmHg with transition from lying flat to standing.
- Electrocardiogram (ECG):
  - Rhythm: Sinus versus non-sinus:
    - Sinus rhythm: P waves axis compatible with sinus node origin (0° to 90°).
    - P wave in front of every QRS complex.
    - Constant P–QRS relationship.
  - Junctional escape rhythm (may be seen with significant sinus bradycardia especially during sleep).
  - Second- or third-degree atrioventricular block (AVB): Long QT interval may cause 2:1 AVB.
  - Compare with previous ECG if available.
- Electrolytes: Calcium, potassium.

Management

- Symptomatic sinus bradycardia is uncommon in children. In most cases cardiac-specific treatment is not required:
  - Correct reversible causes such as hypothermia, hypothyroidism, medication adverse effect, electrolyte imbalance.
- Consult cardiology in the stable/asymptomatic child with bradycardia that does not appear to be sinus bradycardia.
- Symptomatic child:
  - Ensure stable airway and administer oxygen.

○ Consult cardiology for acute third-degree heart block:

■ Isoproterenol may increase escape rate but may cause ventricular ectopy.

■ The use of transcutaneous pacing is rare in pediatrics and requires sedation and involvement of cardiologist or an intensivist.

■ Placement of a transvenous pacemaker wire may be done in a symptomatic child not responsive to medical therapy and is performed by an experienced cardiologist or intensivist.

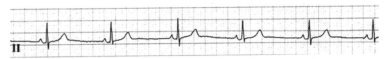

Figure 3-1   Sinus bradycardia.
Courtesy of the Division of Cardiology, Hospital for Sick Children, Toronto.

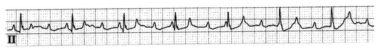

Figure 3-2   Complete heart block.
Courtesy of the Division of Cardiology, Hospital for Sick Children, Toronto.

Tachycardia

- Synonym: High heart rate (HR).
- Definition: Heart rate above the 95th percentile for age (see Table 3-1).

Etiology

- Sinus tachycardia: Response to extracardiac stimuli:
  - Physiologic: Fever, pain, anxiety.
  - Pathologic: Hypovolemia, hypoglycemia, shock, anemia, hypoxia, fluid overload, hyperthyroidism, heart failure, tumors (e.g., pheochromocytoma), pulmonary embolism, medications such as catecholamines and chemotherapeutic drugs (see Table 3-2).
  - Dysautonomia: Chemotherapeutic drugs, chest radiotherapy; paraneoplastic: associated with SVC syndrome, acute lymphoblastic leukemia.
- Tachyarrhythmia:
  - Supraventricular tachycardia (SVT): Primary arrhythmia, intracardiac central venous line.
  - Ventricular tachycardia (VT): Medication, electrolyte disturbance (hypokalemia, hyperkalemia, hypomagnesemia, hypocalcemia), cardiomyopathy, myocarditis, ischemia, hypoxia, acidosis.

Assessment

- Initial assessment: ABC—Airway, Breathing, Circulation.
- Does the ECG rate/rhythm correspond to the cardiac auscultation?
  - Take note of distant heart sounds or a pericardial friction rub that may suggest a pericardial effusion.
- Could an underlying illness explain the tachycardia?
  - Sinus tachycardia versus tachyarrhythmia.
- Is the patient in shock?
  - Weak pulses, inadequate perfusion, altered mental status, decreased urine output.
  - Hypotension is a late sign and signals decompensated shock.

- ECG assessment:
  - Rhythm: sinus versus non-sinus, regular or irregular rhythm.
  - P, QRS, T axis, morphology and interval duration.
  - P–QRS association.
  - Supraventricular tachycardia (SVT):
    - Heart rate: Above the maximum sinus rate but can be within normal limits.
    - Discordant with the physiologic state of the child.
    - HR does not vary, or varies minimally with changes in child's state.
    - P wave:
      - When visible may have an abnormal morphology and or axis.
      - May be hidden in the preceding T wave.
      - Usually fixed P–QRS association.
    - QRS complex:
      - Narrow: Duration is within normal limits for age.
      - Morphology: Often the same as in sinus rhythm; compare with previous ECG if available.
      - QRS duration or morphology may appear different if conduction is abnormal.
    - T wave: Appearance may be normal if conduction is normal.
    - Types of SVT: Atrial ectopic tachycardia, atrial flutter, atrioventricular reentry tachycardia (AVRT), atrioventricular nodal reentry tachycardia (AVNRT), atrial fibrillation, permanent junctional reciprocating tachycardia (PJRT), sinus reentry tachycardia.
  - Ventricular tachycardia (VT):
    - Heart rate is usually above normal.
    - P wave: Typically there is atrioventricular dissociation (look for artifacts distorting the T waves).

- QRS complex:
  - □ "Wide" (above the normal QRS duration for age) − 80 ms is "wide" in a newborn.
  - □ There may be capture beats (ventricle is captured by a sinus beat resulting in a narrow QRS) or *fusion beats* (ventricle is partially depolarized by the sinus beat and partially by the ventricular ectopic beat resulting in a QRS with a mixed appearance).
  - □ When present these findings are pathognomonic for VT.
- T wave:
  - □ T–QRS wave axis > 90.
  - □ More than three consecutive wide QRS complexes define VT.
  - □ Sustained VT: If the run is longer than 30 seconds.
  - □ Incessant tachyarrhythmia: More than 10% of the rhythm per 24 h spent in arrhythmia.
- An important differential of VT is an artifact.
○ "Wide" versus "narrow" QRS tachycardia.
- Electrolytes, acid–base status.
- Chest X-ray:
  ○ Enlargement of the cardiac silhouette may suggest cardiac dysfunction or pericardial effusion.
  ○ Pleural effusions may be seen with a pericardial effusion in a patient with volume overload.
  ○ Position of central venous line.

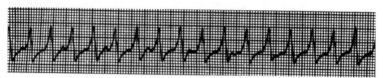

Figure 3-3   Wide QRS tachycardia.
Courtesy of the Division of Cardiology, Hospital for Sick Children, Toronto.

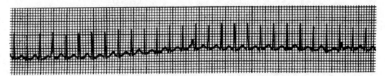

Figure 3-4   Narrow QRS tachycardia.
Courtesy of the Division of Cardiology, Hospital for Sick Children, Toronto.

Management (see Figure 3-5)

- Stable sinus tachycardia:
  - Treatment of potential underlying causes: Restore volume status, treat infection, hypoglycemia, and correct electrolyte abnormalities.
  - Echocardiography (timing depends on clinical course):
    - Exposure to cardiotoxic drugs, cardiomegaly, abnormal ECG, fever or infection not responding to usual treatment, previous cardiac dysfunction/pericardial effusion.
    - Unexplained sinus tachycardia.
- Stable tachyarrhythmia:
  - Adjust central venous line if arrhythmia is associated with recent placement of line or change in position on chest X-ray.
  - Ensure appropriate venous access.
  - Cardiology consultation should be obtained. Treatment and diagnostic options include adenosine, overdrive pacing, or other antiarrhythmic therapy.
  - A stable wide complex tachycardia warrants immediate cardiology consultation.
- Unstable tachycardia:
  - Urgent cardiology consultation.
  - Follow PALS guidelines to restore sinus rhythm and adequate hemodynamics.

○ Keep in mind and treat potential comorbidities contributing to the clinical picture:

- Myocarditis/cardiomyopathy—impending shock (see Shock).
- Pericardial effusion (see Pericardial Effusion).
- Electrolyte abnormalities.
- Acidosis.

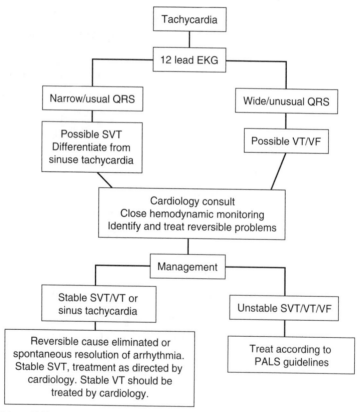

Figure 3-5

Algorithm for the management of tachyarrhytimias.

Shock

- Multifactorial syndrome resulting in inadequate tissue perfusion and cellular oxygenation to meet metabolic needs.
- Among patients with septic shock admitted to PICU, there is a high prevalence of children with oncologic illnesses.
- Cases of septic shock in which the shock state is not reversed often progress to multiorgan system failure, with mortality directly related to the number of organs involved.

Etiology

- Hypovolemic: Dehydration (diabetes insipidus, diabetes mellitus, vomiting, diarrhea), bleeding, third spacing.
- Distributive: Sepsis, anaphylaxis.
- Cardiogenic:
  - LV failure (predominantly):
    - Decompensated cardiomyopathy.
    - Acute cardiotoxicity of chemotherapeutic drugs.
    - Acute myocardial infarction (rare in children).
  - Biventricular failure: Cardiotoxicity, untreated tachyarrhythmia.
  - RV failure (predominantly): Pulmonary hypertension is most common reason in children.
- Obstructive: Cardiac tamponade, massive pulmonary embolism, pulmonary hypertensive crisis, tension pneumothorax.
- Endocrine: Relative adrenal insufficiency, hypothyroidism, hyperthyroidism.

Diagnosis

- Rapid diagnosis and intervention, based on *the rapid cardiopulmonary evaluation*, are essential for reversal of the physiologic disturbances and for favorable outcome:
  ○ Airway patency and stability—need for tracheal intubation?
  ○ Adequacy of ventilation and oxygenation:
    ■ Respiratory rate and effort, air entry: Grunting suggests air space disease (pneumonia) or pulmonary edema.
    ■ Color/noninvasive arterial saturation (Spo_2).
  ○ Circulatory status:
    ■ Heart rate is typically high.
    ■ Assessment of peripheral perfusion and end-organ function:
      □ Peripheral pulses, capillary refill time, skin temperature and color, urine output, level of consciousness and anxiety.
      □ Blood pressure: Hypotension is a late sign and represents decompensated shock.
    ■ Liver size and jugular venous pulse.
- The rapid cardiopulmonary evaluation should be repeated throughout the resuscitation process and is used to assess response to treatment measures and to alter management.
- A careful physical examination should be performed while the first resuscitation measures are under way to determine the possible causes of shock.
- Investigations should not delay initial interventions (Table 3-3).

Table 3-3 Usual investigations in shock.

Lab Tests	Additional Tests
CBC with differential	CXR
ABG, electrolytes (sodium, potassium, chloride), glucose, urea, and creatinine	Abdominal CT (if etiology is not obvious and patient is stable enough for the procedure)
LFTs	EKG
Amylase/lipase	Nasogastric suction (if etiology is not obvious)
Fibrinogen/fibrin split products	Consider echocardiogram based on the preceding information.
Lactate	
Cardiac enzymes	
Venous and arterial blood gases	
Toxicology screen	
Urinalysis, urine culture, urine gram stain	
Blood cultures	
Sputum cultures	
Body fluids cultures (if collections present)	

Differential Diagnosis (see Table 3-4)

The first resuscitation measures are appropriate for all types of shock. The response to them adds useful data for the differential diagnosis.

Table 3-4 Differential diagnosis in shock.

	Hypovolemic	Cardiogenic LV Failure	Cardiogenic Tachyarrhythmia	Obstructive Pneumothorax	Obstructive Tamponade	Septic Early	Septic Late
RR	↑	↑	Normal	↑	Normal	↑	↑
A/E	Normal	↓/Crackles	Normal	↓↓ Unilateral	Normal	Normal/Pn	Crackles/Pn
R/D	None	Orthopnea, grunting	None	Grunting		None	Grunting
Pattern	Hyperpnea		None		Hyperpnea	Hyperpnea, grunting**	
HR	↑	Normal/↑	↑↑*	Normal/↓	↑	↑	↑
Precordium	Normal	Normal/↑	↑↑*	Normal/↓	↓↓	→	↑
Pulses	→	→	→	Normal/↓	Normal/↓	↑	↓
CRT	→	↑	→	→	↑↑	Brisk	→
Skin	Pale, cold, dry	Pale, cold, sweaty	Pale, cold, sweaty	Pale/cyanosis	Pale	Hyperemic, warm, purpura	Cold, purpura
U/O	↓	↓	→	↓	↓	Normal	→
Liver/JVP	Normal/↓	Normal/↑	Normal	Normal/↓	↑↑	Normal	↑
SpO₂	Normal	Normal/↓	Normal	Normal/↓	Normal/↓	Normal	↓
Other clinical	Dehydration	Gallop		Pulsus paradous	Pulsus paradous	Fever	Fever
CXR—lung	Normal	PE	Normal	Dx	Normal	Normal/Dx	ARDS
CXR—heart	Small	Large	Normal/Large	Shifted	Normal/Large	Normal	Normal/Large
EKG	NSR	Abnormal	Dx	Abnormal	Abnormal/Dx	Normal	Norm/Abnormal
Response to fluids	Improve	↑ Liver, PE/ improve	Improve/↑ liver	Improve#	±Improve#	Improve	Improve/ ↓SpO₂/↑ Liver

NOTES: *Well above maximum sinus rate for age **If consolidation present #If hypovolemia present

A/E = air entry; ARDS = acute respiratory distress syndrome; CRT = capillary refill time; Dx = diagnostic; JVP = jugular venous pressure; LV = left ventricle; PE = pulmonary edema; Pn = pneumonia; R/D = respiratory distress; U/O = urine output

Management

- Before an etiology is determined, treatment of shock must be initiated.
- Early goal-directed resuscitation using clinical end points:
  - Normalization of HR.
  - CRT < 2 seconds.
  - Normal pulses with no differential between peripheral and central pulses.
  - Warm extremities.
  - U/O > 1 cc/kg/h.
  - Normal mental status.
- ABC:
  - Ensure secure airway.
  - Administer oxygen therapy.
  - Support ventilation: CPAP, positive pressure ventilation (bag and mask or following intubation):
    - Reduces respiratory effort.
    - Improves ventilation and oxygenation.
    - Decreases LV preload and afterload.
    - Positive pressure ventilation can have negative effects on RV afterload and cardiac output if high pressures are used.
    - Rapid sequence intubation can precipitate cardiac arrest, and mechanical ventilation can be deleterious in certain situations such as cardiac tamponade or tension pneumothorax.
  - Fluids:
    - Initially 20 cc/kg bolus of crystalloid over 5–10 minutes is indicated in suspected septic or hypovolemic shock. 40–60 cc/kg, sometimes more, may be required in septic shock.
    - Liver size is another helpful sign of adequate fluid resuscitation. Hepatomegaly indicates fluid overload.

- If cardiogenic shock is more likely, administration of fluids should be done cautiously with frequent reevaluation.
- In obstructive shock, fluid management must be cautious; may transiently improve hemodynamics but can be also deleterious if excessive. The mainstay of the treatment is urgent correction of the primary cause.
  - ○ Vasoactive drugs/inotropes should typically be used in volume-loaded patients with persistent evidence of hypoperfusion and in patients with suspected cardiogenic shock:
    - Dopamine is usually the first-line agent.
    - Use epinephrine and norepinephrine when refractory to dopamine.
    - Vasopressin—extremely low systemic vascular resistance despite norepinephrine.
    - Hypovolemic and obstructive shock should not require inotropic support once the primary cause has been addressed.
- Antibiotics: Critically important in patients in shock and should be administered early in oncologic patients who are immunocompromised and may have indwelling catheters.
- Other supportive measures:
  - ○ Steroids in septic shock: Catecholamine resistance and suspected or proven adrenal insufficiency; avoid the prolonged use of steroids in severely immunocompromised patients due to the risk of fungal infections.
  - ○ Sedation in patients requiring intubation and mechanical ventilation.
  - ○ Intravenous immunoglobulines (IVIG): unclear.

   ○ ECMO: Refractory pediatric septic shock and/or respiratory failure that cannot be supported by conventional therapies.

Pericardial Effusion

- Common cardiac complication in oncology patients, and may be a sign of cardiotoxicity of a chemotherapeutic agent or effect of the primary disease.
- Pericarditis: Inflammation of the pericardial layers.
- Pericardial effusion: Accumulation of fluid in the pericardial sac.
- Cardiac tamponade: Accumulation of fluid under high pressure in the pericardial sac compromising cardiac filling and cardiac output.

Etiology

- Malignancy: Lymphomas.
- Cardiotoxicity from chemotherapy or radiation (see Table 3-2).
- Uremia.
- Hypothyroidism.

Assessment

- Fever.
- Chest pain: Typically sharp, pleuritic, increasing when recumbent and diminished when leaning forward.
- Pericardial friction rub:
  - ○ Pathognomonic when present.
  - ○ Heard better during expiration, in upright position with the patient leaning forward.

- Dyspnea (respiratory distress): Not a common clinical feature in the absence of cardiac tamponade, pneumonitis or significant pleural effusion.
- Hemodynamic impairment: Pallor, decreased peripheral perfusion, weak and rapid pulses, distended jugular veins, hypotension, pulsus paradoxus, narrow pulse pressure, quiet precordium, distant cardiac sounds:
  - Pulsus paradoxus: Decrease of systolic blood pressure greater than 10 mmHg during inspiration.
  - Beck's triad in cardiac tamponade: jugular distention, hypotension, and muffled cardiac sounds.

Investigations (see Table 3-5)

- At least 50 % of the patients with symptomatic pericardial effusion and malignancy have a nonmalignant cause:
  - Radiation.
  - Opportunistic infections (including TB and fungal).
  - Lymphatic obstruction.
  - Idiopathic.
- Myocardial dysfunction may also be present.

Management

- Asymptomatic patients should be followed by serial echocardiography:
  - Avoid excessive diuretics.
  - Pericardiocentesis may be required for diagnostic purposes.
- Symptomatic patients:
  - ABC.
  - Administer oxygen.
  - Raise the head of the bed.

Table 3-5 Clinical, electrocardiographical, and radiological features of pericardial effusion.

	Pericarditis	Pericardial Effusion	Cardiac Tamponade
Clinical	Chest pain, pericardial rub, dyspnea	Same as P only more dyspnea	Severe dyspnea, Kussmaul sign, decreased peripheral perfusion, hypotension, pulsus paradoxus, Beck's triad
EKG	PR segment depression, ST segment elevation, T wave abnormalities	Same as P + low voltage QRS + electrical alternation with large effusions	Same as for PE
CXR	Unchanged	Blunting of the pericardio-phrenic sinuses, enlargement of the cardiac silhouette (coeur en carafe) with large effusions, normal pulmonary, vascular markings	Same as for pericardial effusion + normal/decreased PVMs + hepatomegaly
Echo	Small rim of pericardial fluid or none	Variable amount of pericardial fluid (even large)	Variable amount of pericardial fluid (even moderate)
	Systolic and diastolic function—normal if no myocardial involvement	Systolic and diastolic function—same as for pericarditis	Systolic and diastolic impairment
Labs	Positive inflammatory markers	Depend on etiology; inflammatory markers may be negative	Same as PE

○ Ensure adequate venous access.
○ Avoid sedation and excessive changes in volume status.
○ If there is symptomatic hypotension administer 5 cc/kg NS bolus.
○ Pericardiocentesis should be arranged emergently.

Congestive Heart Failure

- Congestive heart failure is an important consideration in oncologic patients with the effects of cardiotoxic drugs presenting acutely or in long-term follow-up.
- It is of critical importance to do the following:
  ○ Identify and modify risk factors prior to initiating therapy.
  ○ Institute close cardiovascular monitoring before, during, and in follow-up.
  ○ Minimize the side effects of the therapy.
- The decision to change the chemotherapy needs to balance the goals of achieving remission and of avoiding cardiac morbidity.

Risk Factors (see Table 3-2)

- History of preexisting cardiovascular disorders.
- Prior anthracycline chemotherapy.
- Chemotherapeutic agent.
- Cumulative dose (anthracyclines, mitomycin).
- Total dose administered during a day or a course (cyclophosphamide, ifosfamide, carmustine, fluorouracil, cytarabine).
- Rate of administration (anthracyclines, fluorouracil).
- Schedule of administration (anthracyclines).
- Mediastinal radiation.

- Age.
- Female gender.
- Electrolyte imbalances.
- Concurrent administration of multiple cardiotoxic agents.

Clinical Presentation

- Tachycardia: Unexplained sinus tachycardia is an important clinical sign of potential cardiac involvement.
- Hyperactive precordium, cardiomegaly, diminished heart sounds or gallop rhythm, regurgitant murmur, pericardial rub.
- Dyspnea, orthopnea, grunting, fine crackles in lung bases.
- Hepatomegaly, increased jugular venous pressure.
- Dependent edema.
- Peripheral circulation:
  - Low cardiac output failure: Cold extremities, prolonged capillary refill time (CRT), acrocyanosis, weak pulses, narrow pulse pressure, decreased urinary output.
  - High cardiac output failure: Warm extremities, brisk CRT, bounding pulses, wide pulse pressure.

Etiology

- High cardiac output syndrome:
  - Fever/sepsis.
  - Anemia.
  - Thyrotoxicosis.
  - Valvular regurgitation (endocarditis).
  - Fluid overload.

- Low cardiac output syndrome:
  - Cardiomyopathy: Dilated or restrictive cardiomyopathy following exposure to radiation and/or cardiotoxic drugs.
  - Myocarditis: Chemical, radiation, viral, sepsis.
  - Significant pericardial effusion, constrictive pericarditis.
  - Metabolic myocardial dysfunction: Hypo/hyperkalemia, hypomagnesemia, hypo/hypercalcemia, hypophosphatemia, severe metabolic acidosis, severe hypoglycemia.
  - Arrhythmia: Tachyarrhythmias or bradyarrhythmias.
  - Valvular stenosis/regurgitation.

Monitoring for Cardiotoxicity

- Cumulative dose of cardiotoxic drugs.
- ECG.
- Serial echocardiography.
- Radionuclide angiography.

Management

- Acutely symptomatic patients:
  - ABC.
  - Volume restriction and careful diuresis in the setting of volume overload and there is no suspicion of cardiac tamponade.
  - If there is systemic poor perfusion or the development of metabolic acidosis, management should take place in an ICU setting. Consider afterload reduction and inotrope therapy.
  - Avoid sedation.

- Long-term management:
  - Chronic therapy in heart failure should be managed in consultation with a cardiologist:
    - ACE inhibition is used in the setting of mild cardiac dysfunction.
    - Beta-blocker therapy is added with moderate cardiac dysfunction in combination with an ACE inhibitor.
    - Spironlactone and digoxin may also be used in certain patients with chronic heart failure.
    - Fluid restriction may be required in patients with severe chronic heart failure.

References

Adams MJ, Lipsitz SR, Colan SD, et al. Cardiovascular status in long-term survivors of Hodgkin's disease treated with chest radiotherapy. *J Clin Oncol.* 2004;22(15):3139–3148.

Al-Shekhlee A, Eccher MA, Chelimsky TC. Acute paraneoplastic dysautonomia. *Eur Neurol.* 2003;49(1):64–65.

Barutcu I, Sezgin AT, Gullu H, Esen AM, Ozdemir R. Effect of paclitaxel administration on P wave duration and dispersion. *Clin Auton Res.* 2004; 14(1):34–38.

Carcillo JA, Fields AI. Clinical practice parameters for hemodynamic support of pediatric and neonatal patients in septic shock [in Portuguese]. *J Pediatr (Rio J).* 2002;78(6):449–466.

Dellinger RP, Levy MM, Carlet JM, et al. Surviving Sepsis Campaign: international guidelines for management of severe sepsis and septic shock: 2008. *Crit Care Med.* 2008;36(1):296–327.

Guideri F, Acampa M, Cuomo A, et al. Cardiac dysautonomia in patients with superior vena cava syndrome due to compression by lung cancer. *Int J Cardiol.* 2001;77(2–3):311–313.

Hazinski MF, Zaritsky AL, American Heart Association. *PALS Provider Manual.* Dallas, TX: American Heart Association; 2002.

Irwin RS, Rippe JM. *Irwin and Rippe's Intensive Care Medicine.* 5th ed. Philadelphia, PA: Lippincott Williams & Wilkins; 2003.

Kamath MV, Halton J, Harvey A, Turner-Gomes S, McArthur A, Barr RD. Cardiac autonomic dysfunction in survivors of acute lymphoblastic leukemia in childhood. *Int J Oncol.* 1998;12(3):635–640.

Kruger K. Chemotherapy of sympathicotonic cardiovascular dysregulations [in German]. *Med Klin.* 1971;66(35):1163–1168.

Kutko MC, Calarco MP, Flaherty MB, et al. Mortality rates in pediatric septic shock with and without multiple organ system failure. *Pediatr Crit Care Med.* 2003;4(3):333–337.

Pai BV, Nahata MC. Cardiotoxicity of chemotherapeutic agents. Incidence, treatment and prevention. *Drug Safety.* 2000;22(4):263–302.

Parker MM, Hazelzet JA, Carcillo JA. Pediatric considerations. *Crit Care Med.* 2004;32(11 Suppl):S591–S594.

Rivers E, Nguyen B, Havstad S, et al. Early goal-directed therapy in the treatment of severe sepsis and septic shock. *N Engl J Med.* 2001;345(19):1368–1377.

Veilleux M, Bernier JP, Lamarche JB. Paraneoplastic encephalomyelitis and subacute dysautonomia due to an occult atypical carcinoid tumour of the lung. *Can J Neurol Sci.* 1990;17(3):324–328.

Wilkinson JD, Pollack MM, Ruttimann UE, et al. Outcome of pediatric patients with multiple organ system failure. *Crit Care Med.* 1986;14(4):271–274.

Winkler AS, Dean A, Hu M, Gregson N, Chaudhuri KR. Phenotypic and neuropathologic heterogeneity of anti-Hu antibody-related paraneoplastic syndrome presenting with progressive dysautonomia: report of two cases. *Clin Auton Res.* 2001;11(2):115–118.

Yeh ETH Tong AT, Lenihan DJ, et al. Cardiovascular complications of cancer therapy: diagnosis, pathogenesis and management. *Circulation.* 2004;109: 3122–3131

Yeh ETH. Cardiotoxicity induced by chemotherapy and antibody therapy. *Annu Rev Med.* 2006;57:485–498.

c h a p t e r   4

Endocrine Complications

Sumit Gupta and Stacey L. Urbach

Outline

- Common Abbreviations
- Hyperglycemia
- Hypoglycemia
- Central Diabetes Insipidus
- Adrenal Insufficiency
- Hypercalcemia
- Hypocalcemia
- Approach to the Patient with Multiple Pituitary Deficits

Common Abbreviations

ACTH	adrenocorticotropin hormone
ADH	antidiuretic hormone
BMI	body mass index

Ca	calcium
CRH	corticotropin-releasing hormone
DHEA-S	dehydroepiandrosterone sulfate
DI	diabetes insipidus
DM	diabetes mellitus
FSH	follicle-stimulating hormone
LH	luteinizing hormone
MID	medication-induced diabetes
Na	sodium
SCT	stem cell transplant
SQ	special quantity
TSH	thyroid-stimulating hormone

Hyperglycemia

Etiology

- Occurs in about 10% of patients receiving therapy for acute lymphoblastic leukemia (ALL).
- Related to therapy with exogenous IV dextrose, glucocorticoids, PEG, or *Erwinia* L-Asparaginase, tacrolimus, cyclosporine.
- Most commonly seen during induction chemotherapy (with steroids), sepsis, or stem cell transplant (SCT).
- Risk factors: older age, higher BMI, family history of type 2 DM, trisomy 21.

Clinical Presentation

- Often asymptomatic and noted on routine investigations.
- Severe hyperglycemia: polyuria ± polydypsia, dehydration; rarely acidosis.

- Usually transient and resolves on completion of chemotherapy.
- Long-term significance of medication-induced diabetes (MID) unclear, but may represent predisposition to type 2 DM.

Diagnosis

- Monitor blood glucose premeals if eating, and q 4–6 h when requiring IV fluids.
- Check urine for glucose and ketones when blood sugar ≥ 15 mmol/l (273 mg/dl).
- Monitor intake and output accurately.
- Consider diagnosis of medication-induced diabetes (MID) when two blood glucose levels ≥ 11.1 mmol/l (200 mg/dl).
- If evidence of dehydration/acidosis (tachycardia, Kussmaul respiration, hypotension), monitor blood gases, electrolytes, creatinine, and urea.

Treatment

- Dextrose-free IV fluids when possible.
- Low-concentration carbohydrate diet; ensure caloric intake remains sufficient for patient needs.
- Persistent and/or symptomatic hyperglycemia: consider insulin therapy, preferably with involvement of a pediatric endocrinologist.
- Start with insulin 0.3–0.6 units/kg/day given as subcutaneous injection if eating, and increase as needed to maintain blood glucose 5–10 mmol/l (90–180 mg/dl); see below for dosing regimen.

- Some patients are relatively insulin resistant and require larger doses.
- Consider regimen below but often need to adjust therapy (including dose, number of injections, and insulin type) based on eating pattern:
  - ○ 2/3 of dose given in a.m. before breakfast:
    - ■ 2/3 as intermediate-acting insulin.
    - ■ 1/3 as rapid-acting insulin.
  - ○ 1/3 of dose given in p.m. before dinner:
    - ■ 2/3 as intermediate-acting insulin.
    - ■ 1/3 as rapid-acting insulin.
  - ○ Start with insulin 0.02 units/kg/h given as IV infusion if the patient is unable to eat, or in the presence of acidosis. Use IV glucose infusion as necessary to maintain glucose within normal range; patients are often receiving TPN or high-dose steroids that lead to hyperglycemia and insulin resistance, and do not require additional glucose.
  - ○ Mix 25 units of regular insulin in 250 ml of normal saline (0.9 % NaCl) to make a solution of 0.1 unit/ml.
  - ○ Adjust infusion by 10–20 % increments to maintain blood glucose 5–10 mmol/l (90–180 mg/dl).
  - ○ Monitor blood glucose q 4 h when glucose levels are within target range, and hourly after dose adjustment.
- Higher doses of insulin and additional IV fluids may be needed if evidence of acidosis (involve endocrine team).
- Adjust insulin doses with changes in medication or diet.
- Monitor patients with previous history of MID for hyperglycemia during subsequent cycles of chemotherapy and during intercurrent illness.

Hypoglycemia

Etiology

- Poor intake: nausea/vomiting, anorexia, fasting for procedures.
- Sepsis.
- Adrenal insufficiency.
- Over correction of hyperglycemia.
- Oral purine analogues, e.g. 6-mercaptopurine.
- Younger children at particular risk.

Clinical Presentation

- May be subtle.
- Incidental finding on routine blood work.
- Nervousness, tremor, pallor, headache, diaphoresis.
- Severe hypoglycemia can cause change in level of consciousness and seizures.

Diagnosis

- Repeated blood glucose levels of $\leq$ 2.8 mmol/l (50 mg/dl) warrant complete investigation for underlying etiology.
- Investigations performed during an episode of hypoglycemia include:
    - Glucose.
    - Blood gases.
    - Insulin.
    - Cortisol.
    - Growth hormone (only in a baby or young child).
    - Beta-hydroxybutyrate.
    - Free fatty acids.

- ○ Lactate.
- ○ Ammonia.
- ○ Urine ketones.
- ○ Urine organic acids.
- Consider intervention at blood glucose ≤ 3.2 mmol/l (58 mg/dl) if patient is fasting or unable to eat.

Treatment

- Resuscitation as necessary.
- Oral sugar containing fluids if possible (10–15g of carbohydrate).
- IV therapy if unable to take PO, or if there is a high risk of aspiration.
- Rule of 50:
  - ○ 1 cc/kg of $D_{50}W$, or $(1 \times 50 = 50)$
  - ○ 2 cc/kg of $D_{25}W$, or $(2 \times 25 = 50)$
  - ○ 5 cc/kg of $D_{10}W$ $(5 \times 10 = 50)$
- Address underlying cause of hypoglycemia: stop insulin, treat sepsis, etc.
- Frequent monitoring of blood glucose for response to treatment and for possible rebound hypoglycemia.
- If no cause identified, may require further investigations (e.g., prolonged fast).

Central Diabetes Insipidus (DI)

Definition

- Deficiency of antidiuretic hormone (ADH).
- Destruction of neurons in the supraoptic and paraventricular nuclei of hypothalamus, infundibulum, or posterior pituitary.

Etiology

- Often present at diagnosis of germinoma or Langerhans cell histiocytosis (LCH).
- Common operative complication of therapy for craniopharyngioma.
- Occasionally associated with leukemia/lymphoma due to infiltration, hemorrhage, thrombosis, or infection.

Clinical Presentation

- Polyuria (> 4 cc/kg/h urine).
- Polydipsia: Only if thirst mechanism is intact.
- Hypernatremia, dehydration: If unable to compensate with free water intake (NPO, cognitive delay, young age).

Diagnosis

- Accurate intake and output.
- Urine specific gravity measurements with each void, or hourly if urinary catheter in place.
- Serum sodium, plasma/urine osmolality.
- Very suggestive when evidence of polyuria, urine osmolality < 300 mOsm/kg, urine SG < 1.005, serum sodium > 143 mmol/l, and plasma osmolality > 295 mOsm/kg.
- Water deprivation test (with trained medical supervision): When the diagnosis is unclear or if there is a potential for nephrogenic or psychogenic cause.
- Measure hormones of anterior pituitary as DI is commonly associated with anterior pituitary dysfunction:
  - Thyroid hormone   TSH and free T4
  - ACTH   morning cortisol

    ○ Gonadotropins   LH and FSH if in pubertal age range

    ○ Growth hormone   IGF1, GH stimulation testing if necessary

Therapy

- Manage with support of endocrine team.
- Strict attention to intake, output, and urine SG.
- Monitor serum sodium q 4 h initially.
- Maintain balance between intake and output.
- Allow free access to water if the patient has normal thirst and is tolerating oral intake.
- If the patient requires IV fluids, manage with replacement of insensible losses (400 ml/m^2/day) + urine output using 0.9 % saline or 0.45 NS depending on sodium level.
- Once diagnosis established, use DDAVP therapy.
- Starting doses (treat younger children with lower end of dose range):
  - ○ 0.25–0.5 mcg subcutaneous.
  - ○ 2.5–5 mcg intranasal.
  - ○ 25–50 mcg orally.
- Subsequent doses are adjusted based on response, but are generally required BID to TID.
- Until patient is established on regular schedule of medication, further doses should be given only when evidence of "breakthrough," as suggested by:
  - ○ Urine volume ≥ 4 cc/kg/h.
  - ○ Urine SG ≤ 1.005.
  - ○ Na ≥ 140 mmol/l.
- Allow patient to regulate fluid intake by drinking whenever possible.

- Frequency of sodium measurements can be decreased once patient is on stable regimen of fluids and DDAVP (initially once daily and then even less frequently once levels are stable).

Special Considerations When Diagnosing/Treating DI

- Postsurgical:
  - May have "triphasic" response:
    - Initial DI: Low ADH due to nerve shock, day 1–3.
    - SIADH: Due to release of preformed ADH, lasts 1–14 days.
    - Permanent DI: Once stores are depleted.
  - Patients often receive large volumes of fluid intraoperatively and may excrete large amounts of dilute urine in the postoperative period.
  - Do not diagnose DI without evidence of rising plasma osmolality and rising serum sodium (>145–150 mmol/l) in the immediate postoperative period.
  - 10% of patients may have transient DI.
  - Careful fluid management and monitoring is therefore warranted.
  - Use DDAVP with caution in this group of patients.
  - Initial management in the intensive care unit (ICU) setting is recommended.
- Adipsia:
  - Up to 1/3 of patients with DI may have absent thirst.
  - Need stable daily fluid intake in addition to regular DDAVP therapy.
  - Close monitoring of fluid balance is essential.
- ACTH deficiency leads to free water retention that may mask DI until steroids are initiated.

- Nephrogenic diabetes insipidus:
  - ○ If no/minimal response to DDAVP, no credible cause for central DI, or in situations listed, consider renal cause of DI:
    - ■ Genetic (x-linked, autosomal dominant, autosomal recessive).
    - ■ Chronic renal disease.
    - ■ Metabolic disease (hypercalcemia, hypokalemia).
    - ■ Drug induced (lithium, demeclocyclin).
    - ■ Osmotic diuretics (glucose, mannitol).
    - ■ Amyloidosis.

Adrenal Insufficiency

Definition

- May be primary (adrenal gland) or central (hypothalamus-pituitary).
- Primary adrenal insufficiency is usually associated with deficiency of cortisol and aldosterone.
- Central ACTH insufficiency is associated only with cortisol deficiency.

Etiology

- Suppression of hypothalamic-pituitary-adrenal axis by exogenous steroids.
- CRH/ACTH deficiency associated with intracranial pathology (germinoma, craniopharyngioma, optic glioma), surgery or radiotherapy.
- Adrenal gland injury from trauma/surgery, hemorrhage, infection, or infarction.

Clinical Presentation

- Nonspecific symptoms: Fatigue, malaise, nausea, vomiting, weight loss, headache, hypothermia, change in level of consciousness, hypotension, hypoglycemia.
- Primary adrenal insufficiency presents with above symptoms plus hyperpigmentation, hyponatremia, and hyperkalemia due to aldosterone deficiency.
- Adrenal crisis: Acute deterioration in clinical condition and may manifest as shock, metabolic acidosis, and severe electrolyte disturbance (hyponatremia, hyperkalemia).
- Increased level of suspicion in patients who have recently received course of steroids.

Diagnosis

- Electrolytes, creatinine, renin (elevated with aldosterone deficiency).
- Cortisol level (preferably before 8 a.m.).
- DHEA-S level may be used in postadrenarchal (greater than Tanner 2 pubic hair) children.
- Consider ACTH stimulation test (standard or low dose) if random cortisol or DHEA-S level low:
  - Standard dose: Give 250 mcg of cortrosyn IV.
  - Measure cortisol level at 0 and 60 minutes.
  - Low dose: Give 1 mcg of cortrosyn IV.
  - Measure cortisol level at 0 and 30 minutes.
  - Peak cortisol > 500 nmol/l (18.1 μg/dl) on either test consistent with adrenal sufficiency.
- Some evidence to suggest that low-dose test is more sensitive for central ACTH deficiency, but is technically more difficult to do.

- Unable to assess hypothalamic-pituitary-adrenal axis while receiving glucocorticoids.
- Unable to assess recent onset central ACTH deficiency with ACTH stimulation test, since adrenal glands take time to atrophy after hypothalamic/pituitary injury.
- Normal adrenal glands will respond appropriately to even low-dose ACTH for a number of weeks.
- If high level of suspicion and evidence of clinical deterioration, obtain blood for random cortisol level and initiate therapy immediately.
- If central ACTH deficiency is suspected, assess for deficiency of other anterior and posterior pituitary hormones (see section on DI).

Therapy

- For severe illness or adrenal crisis give hydrocortisone 100 mg/m^2 IV immediately, and then 25 mg/m^2 IV q 6 h.
- Fluid resuscitation with 0.9% saline ± glucose as necessary.
- Correction of hyperkalemia as necessary.
- Maintenance hydrocortisone: 10 mg/m^2/day for central ACTH deficiency, 10–12 mg/m^2/day PO for primary adrenal insufficiency:
  - Young children—3 divided doses.
  - Older children—2 divided doses.
- During intercurrent illness, such as fever/neutropenia, and during admissions for chemotherapy, increase hydrocortisone dose by 3 fold (aim for dose of 30–40 mg/m^2/day PO/IV).
- As patient improves, the dose can be reduced back to baseline over 2–3 days without prolonged taper (e.g.,

1st and 2nd day triple dose, 3rd day double dose, 4th day baseline dose).

- Fludrocortisone 0.05–0.2 mg/day PO divided BID for treatment of mineralocorticoid deficiency (low sodium, high potassium, high renin, low aldosterone).

Hypercalcemia

Introduction

- Occurs in 0.4–0.7% of all pediatric malignancies.
- Seen with hematologic malignancies and solid tumors.
- May be present at diagnosis or during any stage of therapy.

Etiology

- Bone and bone marrow invasion.
- Immobilization.
- Excess ingestion of vitamin D or calcium.
- Thiazide diuretics.
- Paraneoplastic syndrome with release of PTH-related peptide (PTHrp).
- ATRA therapy.
- Subcutaneous fat necrosis, granulomatous disease.
- Adrenal insufficiency.

Clinical Presentation

- Symptoms/signs may be subtle and poorly defined.
- Cardiac: Short QT segment, arrhythmias.
- GI: Nausea/vomiting, constipation, pancreatitis.

- CNS: Lethargy, hypotonia, psychiatric manifestations.
- Renal: Polyuria, nephrocalcinosis, nephrolithiasis, nephrogenic diabetes insipidus, renal failure.

Diagnosis

- Often diagnosed during routine laboratory investigations.
- Symptoms/signs are nonspecific; therefore, maintain high level of clinical suspicion.
- Ca, PO_4, Mg, PTH, ALP, electrolytes, albumin, creatinine, urea, 25-OH vitamin D, 1,25-$(OH)_2$ vitamin D.
- Urine Ca/creatinine ratio.
- Measure ionized calcium if serum albumin or pH abnormal.
- PTHrp may be measured if paraneoplastic syndrome suspected.
- Renal ultrasound to assess for nephrocalcinosis.
- X-rays if clinically indicated (e.g., bone pain).

Therapy

- Acute resuscitation as necessary.
- Calcium levels are sensitive to blood taking technique; confirm abnormal findings in stable patients before initiating aggressive therapy.
- Remove sources of calcium and vitamin D (oral and IV).
- Ensure adequate hydration status.
- Consider ICU monitoring if abnormal ECG, mental status changes, or renal failure.
- In patients with serum calcium $\geq$ 2.9 mmol/l (11.6 mg/dl) or between 2.7 and 2.9 mmol/l (10.8–11.6 mg/dl) with symptoms, proceed as described below:
  ○ Cardiac monitor.

- ○ Hydration with intravenous infusion of 0.9% saline at 1.5–2 times maintenance.
- ○ Establish a good state of hydration, then give furosemide 0.5–1 mg/kg/dose IV (increase renal calcium excretion).
- ○ If the serum calcium remains above 2.9 mmol/l (11.6 mg/dl) 4–6 hours after first dose, a second dose of furosemide can be given.
- • For severe/persistent hypercalcemia, endocrine involvement is highly recommended; also consider:
  - ○ Bisphosphonates: Inhibit osteoclast action leading to decreased bone resorption (effect in 1–3 days and often prolonged):
    - ■ Pamidronate 0.5 mg/kg/day given as IV infusion over 4 h (may repeat after 1 week).
    - ■ Zolendronate 0.01–0.02 mg/kg given as IV infusion over 20 minutes (single dose).
  - ○ Calcitonin: Inhibits bone resorption and increases renal calcium excretion (rapid but temporary effect). Dose: 2–4 IU/kg subcutaneously q 6 h × 3 doses only.
  - ○ Dialysis.
- • Monitor hydrations status, electrolytes, renal function, and hematologic parameters.
- • Address underlying cause.

Hypocalcemia

Etiology

- • Hyperphosphatemia: Tumor lysis syndrome.
- • Hypomagnesemia: Decreased PTH secretion.
- • Pancreatitis.
- • Hypoparathyroidism: Post thyroidectomy.

- Metabolic alkalosis: Increased protein-bound calcium.
- Large volumes of transfusions with citrated products (binds calcium) including FFP, blood, platelets, leukapheresis.
- Dietary calcium deficiency.
- Malabsorption of calcium.
- Vitamin D deficiency.

Clinical Presentation

- Cardiac—long QT segment, arrhythmias.
- MSK—muscle cramps, tetany.
- Neurological—carpopedal spasm (Trousseau's sign), facial twitch (Chvostek's sign), parasthesias, laryngeal stridor, seizures.

Diagnosis

- Often diagnosed during routine laboratory investigations or during monitoring for tumor lysis syndrome.
- Ca, PO_4, Mg, alkaline phosphatase, electrolytes, albumin, creatinine, urea.
- Depending on clinical situation, consider PTH, 25-OH vitamin D, amylase.
- Urine calcium/creatinine ratio.

Therapy

- Acute resuscitation as necessary.
- Consider continuous cardiac monitoring especially if receiving IV calcium.
- Address underlying cause.

- Avoid correction of hypocalcemia in the setting of hyperphosphatemia unless symptomatic. With aggressive calcium correction patients are at risk for calcium-phosphate precipitation and renal failure.
- Most mild hypocalcemia can be managed without administering IV calcium.
- Never give calcium IM, SC, or as an IV bolus.
- Administer infusion as dilute solution (10% Ca gluconate diluted to 2% solution):
  - 10 ml of 10% Ca gluconate contains 90 mg of elemental calcium (2.25mmol); add 10 ml of 10% Ca gluconate to 40 ml of saline to obtain 2% solution; this dilution contains Ca 0.04 mmol/ml.
- For severe hypocalcemia (convulsions, arrhythmias), start infusion at 0.1 mmol/kg/h.
- For less severe cases (cramps, paresthesia), start infusion at 0.05 mmol/kg/h.
- Adjust infusion q 4 h to achieve Ca > 2 mmol/l (8.0 mg/dl).
- Monitor peripheral IV site for signs of extravasation and burns. A central venous line is preferable for administration.
- Calcium and $NaHCO_3$ should not be given in same IV tubing.
- For persistent/unresponsive hypocalcemia, initiate calcitriol 0.1 mcg/kg/day PO (max 2 mcg/day) until calcium returns to normal range. Dose can then be reduced.
- For less severe/asymptomatic hypocalcemia, give oral calcium $\pm$ calcitriol.
- In the setting of tumor lysis syndrome, exogenous IV or PO calcium is seldom indicated unless the patient is symptomatic. If Ca is given, frequent monitoring of electrolytes and renal function is necessary.

Approach to the Patient with Multiple Pituitary Deficits

Etiology

- Most commonly seen in patients with brain tumors, especially germinoma and craniopharyngioma, but may be present in patients with optic glioma and those treated for medulloblastoma.

Management During Admissions for Illness or Chemotherapy

- Ensure all medications are ordered including steroids, DDAVP, thyroid hormone, estrogen/progesterone or testosterone if appropriate.
- Patients do not usually receive growth hormone while on active therapy, but if they are, this may be held during times of illness.
- Strict monitoring of intake and output.
- With existing DI:
  - Urine specific gravity with each void.
  - Measure serum Na q 4–6 h initially.
  - If requiring IV fluids or alteration of usual PO intake, DDAVP should only be ordered for "breakthroughs" and not usual schedule (see DI section).
- With existing adrenal insufficiency:
  - Increase hydrocortisone dose by 3 fold (aim for 30–40 mg/m^2).
  - If not tolerating PO, use IV hydrocortisone at the same dose.
- Manage with support of endocrine team.

References

Ball SG, Baylis PH. Vasopressin, diabetes insipidus and syndrome of inappropriate antidiuresis. In: DeGroot LJ, Jameson JL eds. *Endocrinology*. 5th ed. Philadelphia, PA: Elsevier-Saunders; 2006:3551–3570

Ghirardello S, Hopper N, Albanese A, et al. Diabetes insipidus in craniopharyngioma: postoperative management of water and electrolyte disorders. *J Pediatr Endo Metab*. 2006;19:413–421.

Hopper N, Albanese A, Ghirardello S, et al. The pre-operative endocrine assessment of craniopharyngiomas. *J Pediatr Endo Metab*. 2006;19:325–327.

Howard SC, Pui C-H. Endocrine complications in pediatric patients with acute lymphoblastic leukemia. *Blood Rev*. 2002;16:225–243.

Kerdudo C, Aerts I, Fattet S et al. Hypercalcemia and childhood cancer: a 7-year experience. *J Pediatr Hematol Oncol*. 2005;27:23–27.

Maghnie M, Cosi G, Genovese E, et al. Central diabetes insipidus in children and young adults. *NEJM*. 2000;343:998–1007.

Mathur M, Sykes JA, Saxena VR, et al. Treatment of acute lymphoblastic leukemia-induced extreme hypercalcemia with pamidronate and calcitonin. *Pediatr Crit Care Med*. 2003;4:252–255.

Nasrallah MP, Arafah BM. The value of dehydroepiandrosterone sulfate measurements in the assessment of adrenal function. *J Clin Endocrinol Metab*. 2003;88(11):5293–5298.

Thaler LM, LS Blevins Jr. The low dose (1-μg) adrenocorticotropin stimulation test in the evaluation of patients with suspected central adrenal insufficiency. *J Clin Endocrinol Metab*. 1998:83(8):2726–2729.

Ziino, O, Russo D, Orlando MA, et al. Symptomatic hypoglycemia in children receiving oral purine analogues for treatment of childhood acute lymphoblastic leukemia. *Med Pediatr Oncol*. 2002:39:32–34.

c h a p t e r   5

Gastrointestinal Complications

Oussama Abla, L. Lee Dupuis,
Debbie Chong, and Simon C. Ling

Outline

- Nausea and Vomiting
- Abdominal Pain
- Constipation
- Diarrhea
- Gastrointestinal Bleeding
- Hepatic Dysfunction
- Hepatic Veno-Occlusive Disease

Nausea and Vomiting

Etiology

- Drugs: Antineoplastic drugs; metronidazole, ciprofloxacin; opiates.

- Cranial irradiation.
- Infections: Viral (e.g., rotavirus, adenovirus, CMV), bacterial sepsis, meningitis, encephalitis, urinary tract infection.
- Gastroesophageal reflux.
- Delayed gastric emptying, intestinal pseudo-obstruction, ileus, severe constipation (e.g., due to electrolyte abnormalities, sepsis, postsurgery, opiate analgesia).
- Intestinal obstruction: volvulus, mass effect from tumor, superior mesenteric artery syndrome, intussusception, acute appendicitis.
- Peptic ulceration.
- Intestinal graft-versus-host disease (GVHD).
- Mucositis.
- Pancreatitis.
- Metabolic abnormality: Acidosis, hypoglycemia, hyperglycemia, inborn error of metabolism.
- Raised intracranial pressure.
- Others: Cyclic vomiting syndrome, migraine, celiac disease, eosinophilic gastroenteritis, etc.

Assessment

- History: Assess severity, frequency, relationship to dosing of antineoplastic or other medications, recent surgery, type of vomiting (bile stained, bloody), associated symptoms (abdominal pain, constipation, diarrhea, fever, headache, weight loss).
- Physical exam: Hydration and hemodynamic stability, vital signs, fever, abdominal tenderness, masses, rebound, presence and quality of bowel sounds, rash (e.g., viral or GVHD), signs of sepsis, meningitis, raised intracranial pressure.

- Investigations: As directed by clinical assessment, may include blood work to identify electrolyte or metabolic disturbance, infectious workup (cultures, virology in blood and stool), imaging (2-view abdominal X-ray, abdominal ultrasound to identify intestinal obstruction or pseudo-obstruction, intussusception, etc.), gastric emptying study, upper GI contrast study (for anatomical abnormalities including superior mesenteric artery syndrome and malrotation), possible upper GI endoscopy (to help make specific diagnoses including peptic ulcer disease, CMV infection, GVHD, eosinophilic gastroenteritis or celiac disease).

Gastroesophageal Reflux (GER)

- Suggested by effortless vomiting, accompanied by water brash and/or heartburn, often worse after eating or on lying down. May be complicated by anorexia, dysphagia, poor weight gain, irritability, arching of the back, hematemesis, or anemia.
- Diagnosis can usually be established from the history and physical examination alone:
  - A trial of therapy is a useful way to determine if a symptom is caused by GER.
  - A 24 hour-esophageal pH probe test is a valid measure of esophageal acidity and may help to confirm the diagnosis or to guide therapy.
  - An upper GI barium contrast study is a poor test for gastroesophageal reflux, but it can be useful to identify anatomical abnormalities including esophageal stricture, hiatus hernia, gastric outlet obstruction, malrotation, or upper intestinal obstruction.

○ Hematemesis, anemia, or excess pain are reasons to consider endoscopy in children with GER; consult with gastroenterology.

- Consider the role of additional pathology that may contribute to reflux, such as delayed gastric emptying, and treat appropriately with domperidone or metoclopramide, and a low-fat diet.

Treatment of GER

- General measures:
  ○ In infants with vomiting a trial of a hydrolyzed or amino-acid-based hypoallergenic formula may be helpful.
  ○ In children > 1 year old, left-side positioning during sleep and elevation of the head of the bed may relieve symptoms.
  ○ Children and adolescents should avoid caffeine, chocolate, and any foods that cause symptoms.
- Drug therapy:
  ○ Ranitidine suppresses acid production but is less effective than a proton pump inhibitor for symptom relief and promotion of mucosal healing.
    ■ 5–10 mg/kg/day PO divided BID (maximum 300 mg/day).
    Or
    ■ 2–4 mg/kg/day IV divided q 6–12 h (max 300 mg/day).
    ■ Antacids (e.g., Maalox) may be used to help achieve symptom control during the first 3–5 days of ranitidine therapy.
  ○ Oral proton pump inhibitor (PPI):
    ■ Lansoprazole: < 10 kg = 7.5 mg PO once daily; 10–30 kg = 15 mg PO once daily; ≥ 30 kg = 30 mg PO once daily before breakfast.

Or

- ■ Omeprazole: 1–2 mg/kg/day PO once/day given half an hour before breakfast (max 40 mg/day, round to the nearest 5 or 10 mg).
- ○ Intravenous PPI:
  - ■ Pantoprazole: 1–1.5 mg/kg/day IV as a single daily dose every morning; max 40 mg/day.
- ○ PPI therapy should be continued for 8 weeks or until symptoms and/or precipitating factors (e.g., mucositis) have resolved, and/or precipitating medications (e.g., steroids) have been discontinued.
  - ■ Should symptoms recur within 1 week of discontinuation of a PPI, therapy should be resumed and continued for a minimum duration of 8 weeks.
  - ■ PPIs may impair methotrexate (MTX) clearance and should not be administered for 48 hours prior to intermediate or high dose MTX (≥ 1 g/m^2). PPIs may be resumed once the MTX serum concentration is below the limit specified by the protocol. Therapy with ranitidine may be substituted during this time. High-dose ranitidine therapy may be required when substituting high-dose PPI.
  - ■ For patients with a G-tube, omeprazole suspension is recommended. Preneutralization with an antacid, for at least 1 week, may help to improve omeprazole bioavailability.

Intestinal Obstruction

- Usually presents with bilious vomiting, abdominal pain, constipation, and tenderness on physical examination.

A palpable abdominal mass may be present in intussusception or tumor compression of the intestine. Superior mesenteric artery syndrome occurs most commonly in children with significant weight loss (or recent spinal surgery) and causes vomiting that can be relieved by lying prone.

- 2-views plain abdominal X-ray may show distended loops of intestine and air-fluid levels. Ultrasound may show intussusception and helps with the diagnosis of acute appendicitis or tumor compression of the intestine. Abdominal CT scan is occasionally required to clarify diagnosis.
- Pediatric surgery should be consulted.
- The child should be placed NPO and nasogastric tube suction considered. Attention should be given to restoration of normal electrolyte acid–base and fluid balance using appropriate intravenous fluids.

Gastrointestinal CMV Infection

- Intestinal CMV infection is often accompanied by signs of disseminated CMV including fever, malaise, pneumonia, hepatitis, retinitis, and thrombocytopenia.
- Diagnosis is suggested by gastrointestinal symptoms and positive CMV antigenemia or polymerase chain reaction (PCR) in blood. However, CMV infection can occasionally be limited to within the intestinal tract, and diagnosis then requires histopathological examination and microbiological testing of endoscopic biopsies.
- Consult with an infectious disease specialist and consider therapy with antiviral therapy including ganciclovir and CMV immunoglobulin.

Ileus, Intestinal Pseudo-Obstruction, Gastroparesis

- Can be difficult to distinguish from acute obstruction requiring surgery and should therefore be managed in collaboration with a pediatric surgeon.
- Imaging may show distended stomach or significantly distended loops of small bowel and/or colon, often with evidence of intestinal gas throughout the length of the intestine, including colon and rectum.
- To rule out obstruction, contrast studies by mouth and/or rectum may be required, in consultation with pediatric surgery.
- Identify causative factors including electrolyte disturbance and sepsis, and treat appropriately.
- Consider domperidone or metoclopramide to improve gastroparesis.
- Consider use of nasogastric tube suction.

Note: As gastrointestinal function may be slow to improve, gradual introduction and subsequent maintenance of feeds using an enteral tube (nasogastric or nasojejunal) may be required.

Antineoplastic-Induced Nausea and Vomiting (AINV)

Pathophysiology

- Antineoplastic agents cause nausea and/or vomiting by precipitating the release of many neurotransmitters (e.g., dopamine, serotonin, and substance P) that bind to receptors within the central nervous system and the gut.
- The mechanism through which radiotherapy causes nausea and/or vomiting is less clear but probably involves the release of transmitters including serotonin

due to cell damage within the gut as well as release of emetogenic transmitters by functioning cells.

- Although certain demographic risk factors that predispose adults to antineoplastic-induced nausea and vomiting (AINV) have been identified, none have been identified in children.

Clinical Presentation

- AINV is classified according to its timing relative to the administration of antineoplastic therapy:
  - ○ Acute phase AINV—During the 24 hours after administration of the antineoplastic agent or radiotherapy.
  - ○ Delayed phase AINV—More than 24 hours after administration of therapy, lasting up to 7 days.
  - ○ Anticipatory AINV—Prior to therapy (a conditioned response based on the patient's prior experience with antineoplastic therapy).
- Patients who receive antineoplastic therapy on multiple consecutive days will have a combination of acute, delayed, and anticipatory AINV.
- Uncontrolled acute phase AINV increases the risk of delayed phase AINV, of anticipatory AINV prior to the next treatment, and further acute phase AINV thereafter.
- Although the goal is to prevent all nausea, vomiting, and retching caused by antineoplastic agents and/or radiotherapy, for practical purposes this means maintaining the number of emetic episodes below two per 24 hours during the acute and delayed phases, limiting the duration of severe nausea to less than four per 24 hours, and completely preventing anticipatory vomiting.

Prevention of AINV During the Acute Phase

- Tables 5-1 and 5-2 describe the expected emetogenicity of antineoplastic regimens (based mostly on adult data).
- The emetogenicity of antineoplastic agents given alone or in combination is determined as follows:
  1. Identify the antineoplastic agent with the highest potential to cause AINV in the combination (see Tables 5-1 and 5-2). Use its rank as a baseline.
  2. Assess the emetogenicity of the other agents in the combination (see Table 5-1).
  3. Assign the combination a rank, by adjusting the base rank (from step 1, above) for the rank of the other agents, as follows:
     a. Rank 0 agents do not increase the emetogenicity of the combination (+0).
     b. Adding one or more rank 1 agents increases the emetogenicity of the combination by one rank (+1).
     c. Adding rank 2 or 3 agents increases the emetogenicity of the combination by one rank per agent to a maximum rank of 5 (+1 × number of agents).
  4. Therefore, the combination emetogenicity rank = base rank + adjustment. Examples are provided in Table 5-3.
- The initial antiemetic regimen for a therapy-naive patient is selected from Table 5-4 using the emetogenicity ranking.
- Dexamethasone may be contraindicated; review each patient's protocol to verify. This is a relative contraindication and may be reevaluated based on patient response.

Table 5-1 Acute emetogenic potential of single antineoplastic agents.

Agent	Emetogenicity (anticipated rate of emesis if no antiemetic given)	Rank
Carmustine > 250 mg/m^2 Cisplatin ≥ 50 mg/m^2* Cyclophosphamide > 1500 mg/m^2* Dacarbazine Mechlorethamine	Very high (> 90%)	4
Carboplatin* Carmustine ≤ 250 mg/m^2 Cisplatin < 50 mg/m^2* Cyclophosphamide > 750 to 1500 mg/m^2* Cytarabine > 1000 mg/m^2 Dactinomycin Daunomycin > 60 mg/m^2 Doxorubicin > 60 mg/m^2 Methotrexate > 1000 mg/m^2 Procarbazine Topotecan	High (60–90%)	3
Amsacrine Busulfan IV Cyclophosphamide ≤ 750 mg/m^2* Cyclophosphamide: oral Cytarabine > 100 to 1000 mg/m^2 Daunomycin ≤ 60 mg/m^2 Doxorubicin ≤ 60 mg/m^2 Epirubicin ≤ 90 mg/m^2 Etoposide ≥ 60 mg/m^2 Etoposide: oral Intrathecal antineoplastic therapy Idarubicin Ifosfamide Imatinib Irinotecan Methotrexate 250–1000 mg/m^2 Mitoxantrone < 15 mg/m^2 Temozolamide Vinorelbine: oral	Moderate (30–60%)	2

Table 5-1 (continued).

Agent	Emetogenicity (anticipated rate of emesis if no antiemetic given)	Rank
Etoposide < 60 mg/m^2 Fludarabine (oral) Fluorouracil Gemcitabine Melphalan Methotrexate $51-249$ mg/m^2 Paclitaxel Thiotepa Vindesine	Low ($10-30\%$)	1
Asparaginase Bleomycin Busulfan Chlorambucil Cytarabine < 1000 mg/m^2 Hydroxyurea Lomustine Mercaptopurine Methotrexate ≤ 50 mg/m^2 Methotrexate: oral Rituxumab Teniposide (oral) Thioguanine (oral) Vinblastine Vincristine Vinorelbine (IV)	Minimal ($< 10\%$)	0

NOTE: * associated with delayed/prolonged nausea and vomiting

Table 5-2 Acute emetogenic potential of radiotherapy.

Radiation Site	Emetogenicity (anticipated rate of emesis if no antiemetic given)	Rank
Total body irradiation	Very high (> 90%)	4
Radiation to upper abdomen	Moderate (30–60%)	2
Radiation to lower thorax, pelvis, or craniospinal region	Low (10–30%)	1
Radiation to head and neck, extremities, or cranium	Minimal (< 10%)	0

- There is only limited safety and efficacy data for aprepitant in children, which is therefore restricted to children older than 12 years, over 40 kg, who are receiving cisplatin *and* can swallow whole capsules. Drug interactions with aprepitant may be problematic, including some antineoplastic agents and dexamethasone (reduce dose by half). A hematology/oncology pharmacist should be consulted regarding aprepitant-drug interactions. Aprepitant is given on the first 3 consecutive days of antineoplastic therapy regardless of the length of the antineoplastic therapy course.

- Antiemetics (except aprepitant) should be scheduled around the clock (i.e., not p.r.n.) each day that antineoplastic therapy is given until 24 hours after the last antineoplastic dose.

- Dosages of oral ondansetron are outlined in Table 5-5.

Table 5-3 Examples of calculation of the emetogenicity of several combination antineoplastic regimens.

Combination Regimen:		Combination Emetogenicity Rank
Etoposide 40 mg/m^2 (rank 1)	+ Methotrexate 100 mg/m^2 (rank 1, adjustment +1) + Melphalan (rank 1, adjustment +0)	2
Daunomycin 40 mg/m^2 (rank 2)	+ Vincristine 1.5 mg/m^2 (rank 0, adjustment +0)	2
Cyclophosphamide 1 g/m^2 (rank 3)	+ Cytarabine 75 mg/m^2 (rank 0, adjustment +0)	3
Carboplatin 500 mg/m^2 (rank 3)	+ Etoposide 75 mg/m^2 (rank 2, adjustment +1)	4
Carboplatin (rank 3)	+ Ifosfamide (rank 2, adjustment +1) + Etoposide 40 mg/m^2 (rank 1, adjustment +1)	5
Carboplatin 300 mg/m^2 (rank 3)	+ Cyclophosphamide 600 mg/m^2 (rank 2, adjustment +1) + Etoposide 60 mg/m^2 (rank 2, adjustment +1)	5

Table 5-4   Initial antiemetic selection based on emetogenicity
of antineoplastic regimen.

Emetogenicity Rank of Single Agent or Combination	Recommended Antiemetic Agents During the Acute Phase
Very high (Rank ≥ 4)	Ondansetron 5 mg/m^2 (max 8 mg) IV or ondansetron PO (see Table 5-4), prechemo, and q 8 h *plus* Dexamethasone* 8 mg/m^2 (max 20 mg/dose) prechemo PO/IV over at least 10 minutes and q 12 h thereafter *plus* Aprepitant[†] 125 mg PO × 1 on day 1, 80 mg on days 2 and 3 (NB. Reduce dexamethasone dose by 50% in children receiving aprepitant.)
High (Rank = 3)	Ondansetron 5 mg/m^2 (max 8 mg) IV or ondansetron PO (see Table 5-3), prechemo and q 8 h *plus* Dexamethasone* 4.5 mg/m^2 (max 8 mg/dose) prechemo PO/IV over at least 10 minutes and once daily thereafter
Moderate (Rank = 2)	Ondansetron 5 mg/m^2 (max 8 mg) IV or ondansetron PO (see Table 5-3), prechemo, and q 12 h thereafter
Low (Rank = 1)	Ondansetron 3 mg/m^2 (max 8 mg) IV or ondansetron PO (see Table 5-3) × 1 prechemo
Minimal (Rank = 0)	None

NOTES:

[†] Use of aprepitant reserved for children older than 12 yrs *and* weighing 40 kg or more.

* Use of dexamethasone may be contraindicated if the protocol prohibits its use as an antiemetic or in patients receiving treatment for brain tumors. This relative contraindication may be reevaluated based on patient response.

Table 5-5 Oral ondansetron dose.

BSA (m^2)	Oral Ondansetron Dose
< 0.3	1 mg
0.3–0.6	2 mg
0.61–1.5	4 mg
> 1.5	8 mg

Treatment of Breakthrough AINV

- Breakthrough AINV occurs when > two vomits or retches occur within 24 hours, or when significant nausea lasts ≥ 3 hours per day and affects the patient's activities.
- Treatment should include:
  - Lorazepam 0.025 mg/kg/dose (max 2 mg/dose) IV/PO/SL q 4–6 h p.r.n. for each emetic episode.
  - Escalation of the antiemetic regimen to that recommended for an antineoplastic regimen of the next highest emetogenicity ranking. For example, ondansetron q 8 h rather than q 12 h for moderate emetogens.
  - Consideration of the addition of dexamethasone or an increase in dexamethasone dose to 8 mg/m^2/dose (max 20 mg/dose) q 12 h if applicable.
- If the above measures fail, substitute granisetron for ondansetron and consider additional antiemetic agents such as metoclopramide or nabilone.

Prevention of AINV During the Delayed Phase

- Ensure delayed phase AINV is identified in patients who have been discharged.
- High-risk groups include children with acute phase AINV, with previous delayed phase AINV, or who have received carboplatin, cisplatin, or cyclophosphamide.

- These at-risk patients should receive oral dexamethasone 4.5 mg/m^2/dose (maximum 8 mg/dose) q 12 h with or without ondansetron during the delayed phase.
- If dexamethasone is required in a patient receiving cranial radiotherapy, 1 mg/m^2/day divided BID PO for 7 days is recommended, followed by a tapering dose.
- Routine provision of antiemetic agents to lower-risk patients should be considered on a case-by-case basis.
- Dexamethasone may be relatively contraindicated; review each patient's protocol to verify.
- Ondansetron is not effective in the delayed phase in patients receiving antineoplastic agents of high emetic risk.
- Delayed AINV following antineoplastic agents of moderate emetic risk may be prevented by either dexamethasone or ondansetron.
- Some patients benefit from the addition of metoclopramide 0.1 to 0.2 mg/kg/dose PO/IV q 6 h (consider giving diphenhydramine to prevent extrapyramidal reactions).
- Antiemetics should be given on a round-the-clock basis until the patient is symptom free for 24 hours and restarted if symptoms reappear. If nausea and vomiting increase or persist despite appropriate antiemetics, reevaluate for other causes of vomiting.

Follow-Up

- Ensure that the patient's primary physician and contact nurse are aware when a patient has experienced breakthrough AINV and what antiemetic regimen has been successful in preventing AINV to help with choice of antiemetic agents for subsequent antineoplastic cycles.

Tips

- In children who vomit despite administration of appropriate antiemetic agents, every effort should be made to exclude other possible causes of nausea and vomiting (other than chemotherapy) as mentioned previously.

Suggested Readings

Antonarakis ES, Evans JL, Heard GF, Noonan LM, Pizer BL, Hain RD. Prophylaxis of acute chemotherapy-induced nausea and vomiting in children with cancer: what is the evidence? *Pediatr Blood Cancer*. 2004; 43:651–658.

Dupuis LL, Nathan PC. Options for the prevention and management of acute chemotherapy-induced nausea and vomiting in children. *Pediatr Drugs*. 2003;5:597–613.

Roila F, Feyer P, Maranzano R, et al. Antiemetics in children receiving chemotherapy. *Support Care Cancer*. 2005;13:129–131.

References

Carmichael J, Keizer HJ, Cupissol D, Milliez J, Scheidel P, Schindler AE. Use of granisetron in patients refractory to previous treatment with antiemetics. *Anti-Cancer Drugs*. 1998;9:381–385.

Dupuis LL, Lau R, Greenberg ML. Delayed nausea and vomiting in children receiving antineoplastics. *Med Pediatr Oncol*. 2001;37:115–121.

Gibbons TE, Gold BD. The use of proton pump inhibitors in children: a comprehensive review. *Pediatr Drugs*. 2003;5:25–40.

Gralla RJ, Roila F, Tonato M. Perugia International Cancer Conference VII. Multinational Association of Supportive Care in Cancer. Antiemetic Guidelines. http://wwwmasccorg/media/Resource_centers/MASCC_Guidelines_Updatepdf. Accessed June 25, 2008.

Hassall E, Israel D, Shepherd R, et al. Omeprazole for treatment of chronic erosive esophagitis in children: a multicenter study of efficacy, safety, tolerability and dose requirements. International Pediatric Omeprazole Study Group. *J Pediatr*. 2000;137:800–807.

Hesketh PJ, Kris MG, Grunberg SM, et al. Proposal for classifying the acute emetogenicity of cancer chemotherapy. *J Clin Oncol*. 1997;15:103–109.

Hesketh PJ. Chemotherapy-induced nausea and vomiting. *New Engl J Med.* 2008;358:2482–2494.

Holdsworth MT, Raisch DW, Frost J. Acute and delayed nausea and emesis control in pediatric oncology patients. *Cancer.* 2006;106:931–940.

Holdsworth MT, Raisch DW, Winter SS, Chavez CM. Assessment of the emetogenic potential of intrathecal chemotherapy and response to prophylactic treatment with ondansetron. *Support Care Cancer.* 1998;6:132–138.

Kaiser R, Sezer O, Papies A, et al. Patient-tailored antiemetic treatment with 5-hydroxytryptamine type 3 receptor antagonists according to cytochrome P-450 2D6 genotypes. *J Clin Oncol.* 2002;20:2805–2811.

Lau E, ed. *Drug Handbook and Formulary 2007–2008 SickKids.* Toronto, Canada: Drug Information Service; 2007.

Rudolph CD, Mazur LJ, et al. Pediatric GE reflux clinical practice guidelines. *J Pediatric Gastroenterol Nutr.* 2001;32:S1–S31.

Scott LJ. Lansoprazole in the management of gastroesophageal reflux disease in children. *Pediatr Drugs.* 2003;5(1):57–61.

Abdominal Pain

Assessment

- History: Location, quality, and timing of pain with respect to recent drugs or surgeries, the primary diagnosis. Association with fever, tachycardia, hypotension, vomiting (bilious), hematemesis, bloody diarrhea, constipation, absence of flatus, jaundice.

- Physical exam: Does the child look unwell? Is there abdominal distension? Presence and quality of bowel sounds? Tenderness, guarding on palpation? Masses, organomegaly. Inspection of the perineum and anus, especially in febrile neutropenic children.

- Pain is the principal symptom of an acute abdomen: consider "Does this child need an urgent operation?"

Etiology and Clinical Presentations

- Surgical emergencies:
  - Appendicitis.

- ○ Intussusception.
- ○ Intestinal perforation, peritonitis.
- ○ Small bowel obstruction.
- Infections:
  - ○ Infectious colitis: e.g., *Clostridium difficile*, *adenovirus*, *cytomegalovirus*, *astrovirus*.
  - ○ Sepsis.
  - ○ Urinary tract infection, pyelonephritis.
  - ○ Pneumonia, pleural effusion.
  - ○ Subphrenic abscess.
- Inflammatory gastrointestinal disorders:
  - ○ Gastritis, gastric/duodenal ulcers: High-dose corticosteroids; increased intracranial pressure.
  - ○ Typhlitis, pneumatosis intestinalis.
- Dysmotility:
  - ○ Constipation.
  - ○ Gastroparesis.
  - ○ Intestinal pseudo-obstruction.
- Hepatobiliary disorders:
  - ○ Cholecystitis.
  - ○ Biliary obstruction: Sludge secondary to TPN, stones; lymphoma, neuroblastoma, rhabdomyosarcoma of the common duct.
  - ○ Hepatic veno-occlusive disease (see page 106), Budd Chiari syndrome.
  - ○ Massive hepatomegaly-related to tumor.
- Pancreatitis.
- Tumor:
  - ○ Abdominal compressive mass.
  - ○ Intra-abdominal tumor rupture/hemorrhage.
- Other:
  - ○ Drug related: vincristine, others.
  - ○ Splenic infarction.
  - ○ Functional abdominal pain.

○ Other disorders unrelated to oncological diagnosis (e.g., Henoch Schonlein purpura, inflammatory bowel disease, gynecological disorders).

Diagnostic Workup

- CBC/diff, ESR, amylase, lipase, AST, ALT, GGT, alkaline phosphatase, conjugated and unconjugated bilirubin.
- Blood and urine cultures.
- Stool cultures, *C. difficile* toxin, virology, occult blood.
- Abdominal X-ray (2-views): Helps identify constipation, bowel obstruction; pneumatosis intestinalis may indicate typhlitis, free air suggesting perforation.
- Abdominal ultrasound/Doppler to identify and define masses, lymphadenopathy, abscess, bowel wall thickening, biliary obstruction, and abnormalities of portal or hepatic venous blood flow.
- Abdominal CT—Primarily for characterization of masses and clarification of their relation to adjacent structures.
- Chest X-ray to identify lower lobe pneumonia that may present as abdominal pain; check for subdiaphragmatic free air indicating intestinal perforation.

Typhlitis

Definition

- Necrotizing colitis of the cecum (and sometimes the ileum and ascending colon), also called neutropenic enterocolitis.

Incidence

- Recently increased to 2.6% among children treated for cancer, due to improved detection of typhlitis with cross-sectional imaging and an increased use of CT scan and ultrasound.

Risk Factors

- Leukemia: Typhlitis develops in one third of children with AML on induction therapy; has been reported in ALL on presentation.
- Solid tumors treated with intensive chemotherapy.
- Immunosuppression due to organ or bone marrow transplant.
- HIV.
- Drug-induced neutropenia.

Etiology

- Bowel wall ulceration due to chemotherapy and severe neutropenia ($\pm$ leukemic infiltration) → secondary local infection due to *Pseudomonas aeruginosa, Escherichia coli, S. Aureus, alpha-Hemolytic streptococci, Clostridium, Candida*, or *Aspergillus*.
- Sepsis-induced hypoperfusion → mucosal ischemia and stasis of bowel contents → further injury to the mucosal lining.

Clinical Presentation

- Right lower quadrant (RLQ) pain/tenderness.
- Fever, nausea/vomiting, diarrhea (sometimes bloody).
- Sepsis without localizing abdominal symptoms.

Diagnostic Workup

- Abdominal X-ray: Decreased gas in RLQ with dilated small bowel loops; free intraperitoneal air after perforation; localized or diffuse thumbprinting.
- Abdominal ultrasound/CT: More sensitive; thickened bowel wall or pneumatosis intestinalis.
- Blood cultures: Positive in 50 % of patients.

Management

- Conservative: In 80 % of cases; IV broad spectrum antibiotics covering gram-negative bacteria and anaerobes. NPO, TPN.
- Consult pediatric surgery.
- Criteria for surgical intervention:
  - ○ Presence of free air.
  - ○ Persistent GI bleeding.
  - ○ Uncontrolled sepsis due to intestinal infarction.
  - ○ Need for vasopressor support or larger volumes of fluid.

References

Avigan D, Richardson P, Elias A, et al. Neutropenic enterocolitis as a complication of high dose chemotherapy with stem cell rescue in patients with solid tumors. *Cancer.* 1998;83(3):409–414.

McCarville MB, Adelman CS, Li C, et al. Typhlitis in childhood cancer. *Cancer.* 2005;104(2):380–387.

Shamberger RC, Weinstein HJ, Delorey M, et al. The medical and surgical management of typhlitis in children with acute myeloid (myelogenous) leukemia. *Cancer.* 1986;57:603.

Pancreatitis

Definition

- Inflammation of the pancreas that can present with only pancreatic edema (mild form) or hemorrhage and necrosis (severe).

Incidence

- 2 % in children with ALL.

Etiology

- Drug induced:
  - ○ Therapy with L-asparaginase: most common.

- o Corticosteroids.
- o Cytarabine.
- o Retinoic acid (ATRA).
- o Arsenic.
- o 6-mercaptopurine.
- o Vinorelbine.
- o Liposomal amphotericin-B.
- Other:
  - o Hypercalcemia.
  - o Infections: Viral, bacterial sepsis, mycoplasma.
  - o Hypertriglyceridemia.
  - o Pancreatic duct obstruction (stones, tumor).
  - o Vasculitis, Henoch-Schonlein purpura, Kawasaki disease, hemolytic uremic syndrome.
  - o Trauma.
  - o Congenital anomalies (pancreas divisum, choledochal cyst).
  - o Renal disease.
  - o Diabetic ketoacidosis.
  - o Idiopathic.

Clinical Presentation

- Most prominent symptoms and signs:
  - o Abdominal pain with epigastric tenderness.
  - o Anorexia.
  - o Nausea/vomiting.
- Other:
  - o Fever.
  - o Gastrointestinal bleeding due to coagulopathy.
  - o Jaundice.
  - o Oliguria.
  - o Electrolyte abnormalities.
  - o Respiratory distress.
  - o Circulatory failure.

Diagnostic Workup

- Serum amylase, lipase. Elevated amylase has poor specificity for pancreatitis and can be raised in many other conditions, including gastrointestinal obstruction, acute appendicitis, intestinal ischemia, and salivary gland disorders.
- Serum electrolytes, calcium, BUN, creatinine, liver enzymes including alkaline phosphatase, GGT, conjugated/unconjugated bilirubin and triglycerides.
- Blood gas analysis.
- Viral studies.
- Abdominal US.
- Abdominal CT in selected cases where US imaging is unsatisfactory and greater anatomical definition is required. CT scan with IV contrast will demonstrate the extent of pancreatic necrosis and help with prognostication in severe cases.

Management

- Supportive: Permanent withdrawal of asparaginase in severe hemorrhagic cases; in mild cases, asparaginase can be resumed once symptoms subside.
- Administer intravenous fluids.
- Nasogastric tube for suction if patient has persistent emesis or an ileus.
- Keep fasting initially. When nutrition support is required, enteral tube feeding should be preferred over TPN. Nasojejunal tube feeding may be better tolerated than nasogastric feeds.
- Carefully monitor glucose, electrolytes, and coagulation parameters.
- Broad spectrum IV antibiotics (such as imipenem or meropenem) may be considered in severe, necrotizing pancreatitis to reduce the risk of sepsis.

- Octreotide (5 mcg/kg/day divided BID) may ameliorate L-asparaginase-induced hemorrhagic pancreatitis, but is not routinely recommended in other causes of pancreatitis.
- Consult pediatric GI and surgery.
- Consider transfer to the intensive care unit if there is respiratory distress, ARDS, circulatory failure, or significant electrolyte abnormality.

Complications

- Pancreatic abscess may require open drainage.
- Acute fluid collection may require only monitoring to document resolution with time, unless pseudocyst develops.
- Pancreatic pseudocyst: Supportive care to allow maturation of the cyst beyond 6 weeks, which facilitates internal drainage. Percutaneous or internal drainage (into stomach) may be effective, requiring US or CT guidance and/or gastroscopy.
- Chronic pancreatitis; pancreatic insufficiency requiring enzyme supplementation.
- Septicemia.
- Hypocalcemia, hyperkalemia, hyperglycemia, acidosis.
- ARDS, circulatory failure, renal failure, DIC.

References

Benifla M, Weizman Z. Acute pancreatitis in childhood: analysis of literature data. *J Clin Gastroenterol*. 2003;37:169–72.

Caniano DA, Browne AF, Boles ET. Pancreatic pseudocyst complicating treatment of acute lymphoblastic leukemia. *J Pediatr Surg*. 1985; 20:452.

Garrington T, Densard D, Ingram JD, et al. Successful management with octreotide of a child with L-asparaginase induced hemorrhagic pancreatitis. *Med Pediatr Oncol*. 1998;30:106.

Sahu S, Saika S, Pai SK, et al. L-Asparaginase (Leunase) induced pancreatitis in childhood acute lymphoblastic leukemia. *Pediatr Hematol Oncol.* 1998;15:533–538.

Steinberg W, Tenner W. Acute pancreatitis. *N Engl J Med.* 1994;330:1198.

Constipation

Introduction

- Defined as a delay or difficulty in defecation, usually accompanied by decreased frequency of stooling and the passage of hard stools with discomfort.
- Incidence of 50% in all cancer patients.
- Quality-of-life disruption.

Etiology

- Iatrogenic: Vinca alkaloids (vincristine, vinblastine, vindesine, vinorelbine), opiates (morphine, hydromorphone, codeine), certain antiemetics (5-HT$_3$ antagonists), antidepressants, calcium-channel blockers, calcium and aluminum-based antacids, phenobarbital and ferrous sulfate.
- Functional: Lack of exercise, low fiber in diet, lack of privacy.
- Secondary: External compression from a pelvic tumor, lumbosacral spinal cord compression, pelvic radiation, surgical disruption of nerve pathways, neurofibromatosis, tethered cord, anal stenosis, Hirschsprung disease, Down syndrome, hypothyroidism, hypokalemia, hypercalcemia, dehydration, malnutrition and cow's milk protein intolerance, celiac disease, depression.

Assessment

- History: Obtain baseline stooling patterns and description; family history of similar problems; current or recent chemotherapy drugs and laxatives; associated symptoms such as anorexia, abdominal pain, soiling; recent viral illness; dietary changes and fluid intake.
- Physical exam: Obtain vital signs; abdominal distention and diffuse tenderness may be present; variable bowel sounds; a palpable stool mass may be felt; acute surgical abdomen in bowel obstruction; avoid rectal examination in neutropenic children.

Complications

- Anorexia, nausea/vomiting, abdominal pain, hemorrhoids and anal fissures.
- Fecal impaction, ileus, bowel obstruction, perforation; delays in treatment of cancer.

Prevention

- Identify children at risk early (e.g., those receiving vinca alkaloids, opiate analgesia) and administer prophylactic stool softeners.
- Maintain toilet routines, provide privacy.
- Increase fiber in the diet (whole grains, fruits, vegetables).
- Increase fluid intake.
- Promote physical activity.
- Good patient and parent education.

Investigations

- Serum electrolytes, calcium, magnesium, glucose.
- Thyroid function tests.
- CBC and differential white cell count.
- Consider celiac disease screen: measure antitissue transglutaminase antibody and total IgA.
- Supine/erect abdominal X-ray may show retained stools or small bowel obstruction.
- Neurological assessment including ankle and plantar reflexes and sensation in lumbosacral dermatomes; consider appropriate imaging of spine and/or brain.

Management

- Infants:
  - Prune, pear, and apple juices can decrease constipation.
  - Lactulose can be used as a stool softener.
  - Mineral oil is contraindicated in infants due to the risk of lipoid aspiration pneumonia.
  - Stimulant laxatives are rarely recommended for infants < 1 year.
- Children:
  - Ensure preventative measures above are in place.
  - Use lactulose to soften stool.
  - In the presence of stool impaction, soften stool with lactulose over several days and then provide stimulant laxative such as Pico-salax, or cleanout with high volume polyethylene glycol preparation (usually requires an NG tube).
  - Effective maintenance therapy can usually be achieved with lactulose, occasionally with addition of senna.
  - Polyethylene glycol provided as PEGFlakes or Miralax are an effective alternative in those children who respond poorly to lactulose.

o Avoid rectal administration (i.e., suppositories and enemas) in neutropenic patients.

o The use of Fleet enemas may be considered in severe cases, in nonneutropenic patients, and at the discretion of the responsible physician.

References

Clinical practice guideline: evaluation and treatment of constipation in infants and children; recommendations of the North American Society for Pediatric Gastroenterology, Hepatology and Nutrition. *J Pediatr Gastroenterol Nutr*. 2006;43(3):.

Selwood K. Constipation in paediatric oncology. *Eur J Oncol Nursing*. 2006; 10:68–70.

Woolery M, Carroll E, Fenn E, et al. A constipation assessment scale for use in pediatric oncology. *J Pediatr Oncol Nursing*. 2006;23(2):65–74.

Diarrhea

Introduction

- Defined as the presence of increased stool frequency and volume or a change to a looser stool consistency.
- Incidence: Occurs in 10 % of patients with advanced cancer and in up to 50–80 % of those receiving irinotecan or 5-fluorouracil (5-FU).
- Severe diarrhea can potentially be life threatening by delaying cancer treatment, due to reduced patient compliance or fluid and electrolyte abnormalities.

Etiology

- Chemotherapy drugs such as irinotecan, topotecan, 5-FU, cytarabine, cisplatin, cyclophosphamide, daunorubicin, methotrexate, leucovorin, interferon and dasatinib.

- Other drugs: Overuse of laxatives/stool softeners, metoclopramide, opiate withdrawal, antibiotics, antacids, antihypertensives, magnesium, potassium or phosphate supplements, herbal supplements.
- Abdominal radiation therapy.
- Infections: Pseudomembranous colitis, viral, bacterial, parasitic or fungal gastroenteritis.
- Typhlitis, severe mucositis.
- Intestinal ischemia.
- Gut graft-versus-host-disease (GVHD).
- Tumors: Neuroblastoma (VIP-secreting), lymphomas, gastrointestinal-stromal tumor (GIST).
- Dietary intolerance: Lactose intolerance, high-fiber food.
- Small bowel bacterial overgrowth.
- Irritable bowel syndrome.
- Pancreatic insufficiency (chronic GVHD, cystic fibrosis, Schwachman-Diamond syndrome).
- Other primary gastrointestinal disease: Celiac disease, cow's milk protein enteropathy, lactose intolerance, inflammatory bowel disease, etc.

Assessment

History

- Onset and duration of diarrhea.
- Description of stool volume, frequency, and composition (e.g., watery, bloody).
- Associated signs: Fever, nausea/vomiting, dizziness, abdominal pain, weight loss (rule out sepsis, dehydration or bowel obstruction).
- Medication profile: Identify any diarrheogenic agent; ask if any drugs taken to control diarrhea.

- Dietary and fluid intake; association of diarrhea with any specific foods.
- Infectious disease contacts, recent travel history.
- Ask about site and stage of cancer and any current or recent treatment (e.g., type of chemotherapy, radiation, or allogenic bone marrow transplant).
- Family history of gastrointestinal or autoimmune diseases.

Physical Exam

- Hydration status; vital signs (R/O postural hypotension).
- Abdomen: Presence of distention, hyperactive or hypoactive bowel sounds, tenderness, guarding, masses or organomegaly.
- Assess perianal skin integrity: Can have severe breakdown due to diarrhea especially after high-dose methotrexate/cytarabine, daunorubicin, or bone marrow transplant.
- Avoid rectal examination in neutropenic patients.

Diagnostic Workup

- Stool for occult blood, cultures (salmonella, *E. coli*, campylobacter, etc.), *Clostridium difficile* toxin microscopy for ova and parasites (cryptosporidium, giardia, ameba), and virology.
- CBC, differential white cell count, electrolytes, BUN, creatinine, celiac screen, viral studies (e.g., CMV).
- If cause remains unclear after history, physical examination, and above tests, then consider imaging with abdominal X-rays and abdominal ultrasound scan for

evidence of partial obstruction, dilated small intestine at risk of small bowel overgrowth, pneumatosis intestinalis and/or bowel wall thickening in typhlitis or other inflammatory bowel disease, or evidence of tumor. Proceed if necessary to upper gastrointestinal series with small bowel follow-through or abdominal CT scan with contrast to further clarify the intra-abdominal pathology.

- Consider 3-day stool collection for measurement of total fat excretion combined with dietary assessment to calculate the fractional excretion of fat.
- Consult pediatric gastroenterology. Consider upper GI endoscopy and/or colonoscopy to identify evidence of mucosal diseases including CMV infection, GVHD, celiac disease, eosinophilic gastroenteritis, or other inflammatory bowel disease. Endoscopic procedures should be avoided whenever possible in children with typhlitis due to the risk of perforation and in children with neutropenia/thrombocytopenia due to the risks of septicemia and/or hemorrhage from biopsy sites.

General Management

- Avoid milk and dairy products if there is evidence of cow's milk protein or lactose intolerance.
- Avoid bulk laxatives, stool softeners, metoclopramide; reduce or withdraw magnesium/potassium/phosphate supplements; stop all herbal products that can cause diarrhea, such as milk thistle, aloe, Siberian ginseng, green tea, coenzyme Q10 and high doses of vitamin C.
- Oral hydration: Increase fluid intake (especially in severe diarrhea, dehydration), encourage clear fluids

such as broth and glucose/electrolyte drinks (e.g., Gatorade, Pedialyte). Give IV hydration in case of persistent vomiting, sepsis, or severe mucositis.

- In case of typhlitis or ileus, keep NPO and provide IV hydration and nutrition (see pages 84–86).

Management of Specific Causes

- Chemotherapy induced diarrhea:
  - Mild: Loperamide.
  - Severe: Octreotide at 10–40 mcg/kg/day IV/SC divided q 8 h.
- Gastrointestinal radiation toxicity:
  - Prevention by reduced dose and field of radiation.
  - Possible benefit from sulfasalazine (40–70 mg/kg/day PO div q 8 h).
  - Symptomatic treatment with loperamide if mild.
  - Octreotide may have a role for more severe secretory diarrhea.
- Infections:
  - Whether or not to treat, and the choice of treatment, depends on the infectious agent and clinical circumstances.
  - Symptomatic *C. difficile* infection should be treated with oral metronidazole, and treatment failures with oral vancomycin.
- Gastrointestinal ischemia or infarction: Consultation with surgery regarding need for, and timing of, laparotomy.
- Pancreatic insufficiency: Supplementation with oral pancreatic enzymes.
- Other:
  - Irritable bowel syndrome may benefit from reassurance, dietary manipulation, psychology input, or

pharmacological treatment in consultation with a gastroenterologist.

○ Other gastrointestinal diseases should be managed in consultation with a gastroenterologist.

References

O'Brien BE, Kaklamani VG, Benson AB. The assessment and management of cancer treatment-related diarrhea. *Clin Colorectal Cancer*. 2005;4(6): 375–381.

Gastrointestinal Bleeding

Etiology

Upper GI Bleeding

- Esophagitis.
- Esophageal varices: e.g., in LCH, abdominal tumors, portal vein thrombosis.
- Gastritis, gastroduodenal ulceration: Stress ulceration, steroids, *Helicobacter pylori*, CMV.
- Swallowed blood from epistaxis or oropharyngeal mucositis.
- Mallory-Weiss tear following chemotherapy-induced emesis.
- Coagulopathy: Hemophilia, thrombocytopenia, DIC.
- Anatomic and vascular anomalies: Hemangiomas, gastrointestinal telangiectasia.
- Malignant disease: Burkitt's lymphoma, lymphoproliferative disease, gastrointestinal stromal tumors, gastric teratoma, pancreatic carcinoma.

Lower GI Bleeding

- Typhlitis.
- Infection: *C.difficile* pseudomembranous colitis, cryptosporidium, fungi.
- Anal fissures, hemorrhoids (e.g., secondary to severe constipation).
- Intussusception (e.g., polyp or tumor as lead point).
- Malignant disease: Burkitt's lymphoma, PTLD.
- Coagulopathy, thrombocytopenia, DIC.
- Meckel's diverticulum.
- Volvulus.
- Hemolytic uremic syndrome.
- Enterocolitis: Necrotizing, radiation.
- Multifactorial.

Assessment

History

- Onset, frequency, and quality of bleeding: Coffee ground vomits, bright red hematemesis, or melena suggest upper gastrointestinal source. Initial repeated nonbloody vomits followed by hematemesis suggests Mallory Weiss tear. Dark red or maroon-colored blood per rectum is suggestive of distal small intestinal source, such as Meckel's diverticulum, or very brisk upper GI source. Bright red blood per rectum comes from the colon.
- Associated abdominal pain, diarrhea, vomiting, fever and rectal pain.
- Signs of hemodynamic instability.
- Assess for bleeding in other areas—epistaxis or mucositis.

- Previous history of bleeding.
- Drug history—steroids, antibiotics..
- Type and site of cancer; recent treatment given (chemotherapy, BMT, radiation), recent surgery or gastrointestinal endoscopy.

Physical Exam

- Assess hemodynamic stability: vital signs, orthostatic BP, capillary perfusion, urine output, mental status to determine severity of bleeding and shock.
- Evidence of bleeding disorder or coagulopathy (e.g., petechiae, purpura), vascular abnormalities (cutaneous hemangiomas, telangiectasias), liver disease (jaundice, spider naevi, palmar erythema, encephalopathy).
- Abdominal exam: Bowel sounds, tenderness, rebound, masses, hepatosplenomegaly.
- Perianal and rectal exam: Rule out anal fissures, hemorrhoids, rectal abscess; avoid rectal exploration in neutropenic patients.

Diagnostic Workup

- CBC, platelets, coagulation studies.
- Plain AXR (two views) for evidence of volvulus, intussusception, typhlitis, necrotizing enterocolitis.
- US abdomen for evidence of liver disease, tumor.
- Infectious work-up if relevant (stools, cultures, virology).
- Passage of NG tube to assess presence of fresh blood in stomach (avoid if portal hypertensive bleeding suspected).
- 99 mTc Meckel's scan if maroon or dark red blood per rectum.

- Upper gastrointestinal endoscopy and/or colonoscopy; usually undertaken following stabilization with medical therapy (below) in order to identify cause and enable intervention to reduce risk of rebleeding. Occasionally, interventional endoscopy is required to stop active bleeding.

Management

- If severe or recurrent bleeding: consult the pediatric gastroenterology and surgical services.
- Clinical assessment and investigations listed above should determine the need for the following:
  - Immediate surgical intervention (e.g., volvulus, Meckel's diverticulum).
  - The appropriateness of awaiting culture and virology results before initiating management.
  - The need for only topical therapy for anal fissure.
  - The need for oral PPI therapy for minor bleeding, due to probable esophagitis, stress ulcer, or steroid-induced gastropathy.
- Correct intravascular volume and anemia appropriately with bolus administration of 0.9% sodium chloride solution, red blood cells, or other blood products as appropriate.
- Optimize coagulation parameters in patients with coagulopathy with infusions of platelets, fresh frozen plasma, cryoprecipitates, or factor concentrates as appropriate to the clinical circumstances.
- If there is severe, acute upper GI hemorrhage without evidence of liver disease or need for acute surgical intervention:
  - Give intravenous bolus dose of pantoprazole followed by continuous infusion (see Chapter 19 for dosage).

- In consultation with a pediatric gastroenterologist, consider the need for early upper GI endoscopy, dependent upon the patient's hemodynamic stability, severity of bleed, and likely etiology. Endoscopy may provide a more accurate diagnosis and may allow therapeutic intervention to stop ongoing bleeding or to prevent rebleeding.
- If there is severe, acute upper GI hemorrhage in the presence of liver disease or portal hypertension:
  - Give intravenous octreotide bolus dose (1–2 mcg/kg IV) followed by infusion (1–5 mcg/kg/h IV).
  - Give intravenous bolus dose of pantoprazole followed by continuous infusion.
  - Provide broad spectrum antibiotic coverage due to the high risk of sepsis following portal hypertensive GI bleeding.
  - Plan for early upper GI endoscopy to enable diagnosis of the source of bleeding (esophageal or gastric varices, portal hypertensive gastropathy, gastric or duodenal ulcer, etc.) and to allow endoscopic treatment to reduce the risk of rebleeding.
- Children with ongoing severe gastrointestinal hemorrhage with hemodynamic instability in spite of treatment with intravenous PPI and octreotide as appropriate should be urgently reviewed by gastroenterology and surgery. Management may require the following:
  - Endoscopy or colonoscopy by a gastroenterologist experienced in the management of acute GI bleeding.
  - Identification of a bleeding source beyond the reach of endoscopy/colonoscopy may be achieved by radio-labeled red cell scan, angiography (possibly with embolization of vessels that feed the bleeding point), or laparotomy (sometimes combined with intraoperative enteroscopy).

- Recombinant activated factor VII (rFVIIa) can be help-ful in severe intractable upper GI bleeding. Usual dose = 90 mcg/kg IV; consult a pediatric hematologist expert in hemostasis.

References

Dewar GJ, Lim CN, Michal Y, et al. Gastrointestinal complications in patients with acute and chronic leukemia. *Can J Surg.* 1981;24:67.

Durbin DR, Liacouras CA. Gastrointestinal emergencies. In: Fleisher GR, Ludwig S, eds. *Textbook of Pediatric Emergency Medicine.* 4th ed. Philadelphia, PA: Lippincott Williams & Wilkins; 1999:1017.

Kurekci AE, Atay AA, Okutan V, et al. Recombinant activated factor VII for severe gastrointestinal bleeding after chemotherapy in an infant with acute megakaryoblastic leukemia. *Blood Coagul Fibrinolysis.* 2005;16: 145–147.

Trepanier EF. Intravenous pantoprazole: a new tool for acutely ill patients who require acid suppression. *Can J Gastroenterol.* 2000;14:11D-18D.

Hepatic Dysfunction

Etiology

- Chemotherapy drugs: Anthracyclines (daunorubicin, idarubicin), vincristine, vinblastine, methotrexate (especially high-dose), 6-mercaptopurine, 6-thioguanine, etoposide, cytarabine, L-asparaginase, busulfan, cyclophosphamide, actinomycin-D and monoclonal antibodies (gemtuzumab).
- Other drugs: Azoles (fluconazole, voriconazole, posaconazole, itraconazole), caspofungin, amphotericin-B, cotrimoxazole, steroids, etc.
- Infections: Viral (hepatitis A, B, C; CMV, EBV, Varicella-Zoster virus, adenovirus, herpes viruses, RSV); bacterial sepsis; fungal (candida albicans, aspergillus).

- Disease related: Hepatic graft-versus-host-disease; HLH; primary tumor (hepatoblastoma) or secondary tumor (leukemic or solid tumor infiltrate).
- TPN-associated liver disease.
- Gallstones.
- Other coincidental liver disease (e.g., nonalcoholic fatty liver disease, a-1 antitrypsin deficiency, autoimmune hepatitis, other metabolic disease).

Clinical Scenarios

- Hepatitis—predominant elevation of transaminases.
- Cholestasis—predominant conjugated hyperbilirubinemia and elevation of GGT or alkaline phosphatase.
- Hepatic veno-occlusive disease.
- Fulminant liver failure.
- Chemotherapy-induced hepatotoxicity:
  - ○ Occurs in 24% of children treated for AML.
  - ○ Usually limited to asymptomatic increase in LFTs.
  - ○ Rarely severe and frequently without clinical consequence.

Diagnostic Workup

- Assess pattern and severity of liver injury by checking liver enzymes, bilirubins, albumin, INR and ammonia.
- Comprehensive review of all medications.
- Virologic serology and PCR, bacterial and fungal septic workup.
- Abdominal ultrasound scan including liver, spleen, and Dopplers to assess diffuse or focal hepatic parenchymal abnormality, bile duct abnormalities including biliary

obstruction, spleen size, lymphadenopathy, evidence of portal hypertension, ascites, other masses.

- Abdominal CT when required following ultrasound scan.
- GI consultation for extended workup for coincidental liver disease and consideration of liver biopsy in rare cases.

Treatment

- Mainly supportive.
- Reduce dose or delay chemotherapy drugs in case of increased conjugated hyperbilirubinemia (anthracyclines, vincristine, HD-MTX, asparaginase).
- Delay HD-MTX if AST > 500.
- During maintenance therapy for ALL, oral doses of 6-MP and or MTX may need to be decreased or withheld for persistent severe elevations of transaminases.
- Ensure INR is optimized with adequate doses of vitamin K, and consider infusions of FFP, fibrinogen, or albumin as indicated.
- Acute liver failure should be managed in consultation with the gastroenterology service and the intensive care unit when appropriate.
- Gallstones obstructing the biliary tree require removal by ERCP and subsequent cholecystectomy. Intravenous broad spectrum antibiotics should be given in the presence of fever.
- Cholestasis and/or biliary sludge related to parenteral nutrition may benefit from oral dosing with ursodeoxycholic acid.
- Treatment of infectious agents with antibiotics and antiviral and antifungal agents as appropriate, in consultation with infectious disease specialist if required.
- Treat HVOD (see pages 106–109).

References

Creutzig U, Ritter J, Zimmermann M, et al. Idarubicin improves blast cell clearance during induction therapy in children with AML: results of study AML-BFM 93. AML BFM Study Group. *Leukemia*. 2001;15:348–354.

Lee WM. Drug-induced hepatotoxicity. *N Engl J Med*. 2003;349:474–485.

Weber BL, Tanyer G, Poplack DG, et al. Transient acute hepatotoxicity of high-dose methotrexate therapy during childhood. *NCI Monogr*. 1987; 5:207–212.

Hepatic Veno-Occlusive Disease

Definition

- Hepatic venous occlusive disease (HVOD) or sinusoidal obstruction syndrome is a clinical syndrome consisting of hepatomegaly, fluid retention, ascites, and jaundice.
- HVOD is a result of disruption of intrahepatic circulation caused by sinusoidal endothelial cell injury and does not require obstruction of the hepatic veins.

Etiology

- HVOD is most commonly described after busulfan, cyclophosphamide, and/or TBI conditioning for hematopoietic stem cell transplant (HSCT).
- Outside of the HSCT setting, HVOD has been associated with administration of cyclophosphamide and roxithromycin; gemtuzumab ozogamicin; dactinomycin and vincristine; dactinomycin, vincristine, and cyclophosphamide; thioguanine; oxaliplatin; 6-mercaptopurine; and cytosine arabinoside.
- The incidence of HVOD as a consequence of gemtuzumab ozogamicin therapy in adults has been estimated to be 3% to 28%.

Precautions

- Risk factors for HVOD such as donor type, recent prior HSCT, high busulfan exposure, and underlying malignant disease have been identified in HSCT patients.
- Risk factors for HVOD that have been identified in patients receiving conventional dose antineoplastic therapy include prior liver disease and radiation.
- Risk factors for HVOD due to gemtuzumab ozogamicin in adults are high-dose, concomitant administration of other hepatotoxins and HSCT within the prior 3–4 months.

Clinical Presentation

- Clinical criteria for diagnosis of HVOD in the HSCT setting have been developed and are conventionally applied to patients with antineoplastic-associated hepatopathy.
- The Jones criteria stipulate that the diagnosis of HVOD requires hyperbilirubinemia (total serum bilirubin > 34 (mol/l) and at least two of the following clinical findings: right upper quadrant pain (tender hepatomegaly), ascites, or weight gain > 5% above baseline.
- Some authors have proposed that, outside of the HSCT setting, the presence of clinical signs and elevation of transaminase concentrations with or without hyperbilirubinemia is sufficient to make the diagnosis of HVOD.
- Symptom onset ranges from 1 to 4 weeks after antineoplastic administration. Elevation in transaminase concentrations may persist for up to 2 months.

Investigations

- Other possible causes of liver impairment must be investigated, such as viral hepatitis and fungal infection.
- A diagnosis of HVOD is made clinically; radiological testing (e.g., ultrasound evidence of reduced hepatic venous flow) may support the diagnosis but is not conclusive.
- Hepatic imaging is useful to rule out biliary obstruction, infection, and malignancy.
- Doppler ultrasound may show reduction of hepatic blood flow.
- Liver biopsy may confirm the diagnosis but is rarely undertaken due to concurrent coagulopathy and thrombocytopenia.

Treatment

- HVOD associated with conventional antineoplastic therapy is usually reversible and does not lead to long-term hepatic impairment.
- In some cases, antineoplastic therapy that appeared to have caused HVOD in one cycle has been resumed, though initially at lower doses with gradual escalation to full doses.
- Administration of oral ursodiol at the first sign of hyperbilirubinemia, even in the absence of other clinical signs of HVOD, may be beneficial.
- Administration of alteplase (tPA), heparin, prostaglandins, or urokinase is not useful and is associated with adverse effects.
- Most patients respond to supportive therapy including fluid and sodium restriction.

- Defibrotide, which has pro-fibrinolytic and antithrombotic properties, may be used in severe cases: 36% response rate, without adverse events.

Outcomes

- HVOD associated with HSCT entails a high risk of mortality. Multiorgan failure is a more common cause of death than liver failure alone.
- Mortality due to HVOD resulting from conventional antineoplastic administration is unusual.

References

Sulis ML, Bessmertny O, Granowetter L, et al. Veno-occlusive disease in pediatric patients receiving actinomycin D and vincristine only for the treatment of rhabdomyosarcoma. *J Pediatr Hematol Oncol.* 2004;26:843–846.

Tack DK, Letendre L, Kamath PS, Tefferi A. Development of hepatic veno-occlusive disease after Mylotarg infusion for relapsed acute myeloid leukemia. *Bone Marrow Transplant.* 2001;28:895–897.

Beltinger J, Haschke M, Kauffmann P, et al. Hepatic veno-occlusive disease associated with immunosuppressive cyclophosphamide dosing and roxithromycin. *Ann Pharmacother.* 2006;40:767–770.

Kallianpur AR, Hall LR, Yadav M, et al. The hemachromatosis C282Y allele: a risk factor for hepatic veno-occlusive disease after haematopoietic stem cell transplantation. *Bone Marrow Transplant.* 2005;53:1155–1164.

Srivastava A, Poonkuzhali B, Shaji RV, et al. Glutathione S-transferase M1 polymorphism: a risk factor for hepatic veno-occlusive disease in bone marrow transplantation. *Blood.* 2004;104:1574–1577.

McKoy JM, Angelotta C, Bennett CL, et al. Gemtuzumab ozogamicin-associated sinusoidal obstructive syndrome (SOS): an overview from the research on adverse drug events and reports (RADAR) project. *Leukemia Res.* 2007;31:599–604.

Senzolo M, Germani G, Cholongitas E, et al. Veno occlusive disease: update on clinical management. *World J Gastroenterol.* 2007;13(29):3918–3924.

c h a p t e r   6

Hematologic Complications

Michaela Cada, Wendy Lau, and Manuel D. Carcao

Outline

- Bleeding Diathesis
- The Coagulation Cascade
- Approach to the Bleeding Patient
- Transfusion Therapy Guidelines
- Transfusion Reactions
- Platelet Refractoriness

Bleeding Diathesis

Etiology of Thrombocytopenia

- Decreased production:
  - Marrow suppression: Chemotherapy, irradiation, infection.

○ Marrow infiltration: Leukemia, neuroblastoma, solid tumors.
- Increased destruction:
  ○ Consumption: Disseminated intravascular coagulation (DIC), common; hypersplenism, rare.
  ○ Immune-mediated platelet destruction: Alloimmunization.

Etiology of Coagulopathy

- L-asparaginase causes reduction in synthesis of procoagulant factors (fibrinogen, factor V, and vitamin K-dependent factors) predisposing to bleeding, and anticoagulant factors (plasminogen, AT, protein C, protein S) predisposing to thrombosis.
- Liver dysfunction: Poor synthesis of multiple clotting factors:
  ○ Hepatotoxicity secondary to chemotherapy, azoles, caspofungin, TPN.
  ○ Infections.
  ○ Hepatic veno-occlusive disease, GVHD.
  ○ Metastatic tumor.
  ○ Biliary obstruction, etc.
- Vitamin K deficiency:
  ○ Decreased oral intake.
  ○ Decreased intestinal absorption.
  ○ Suppression of bowel flora by antibiotics.
- DIC: Inappropriate and excessive activation of blood coagulation leading to consumption of clotting factors and platelets. Seen in:
  ○ Sepsis.
  ○ Acute promyelocytic leukemia (APL), acute myeloid leukemia (AML).

- ○ Acute lymphoblastic leukemia (ALL): esp. T-cell, hyperleukocytosis.
- ○ Metastatic neuroblastoma, rhabdomyosarcoma.
- Other:
  - ○ Renal failure: Uremia +/− loss of protein.
  - ○ Acquired von Willebrand's disease (VWD): Infrequently seen with Wilms' tumor.

The Coagulation Cascade

- Clotting is made possible by a cascade of events involving various coagulation factors and platelets (Figure 6-1).
- All coagulation factors are made exclusively by the liver except FVIII and von Willebrand factor (VWF) → in severe liver failure all factor levels, except FVIII and VWF, are reduced.
- Vitamin K-dependent factors: II, VII, IX, X, protein C and S.
- Coagulation factors have different clearance mechanisms → different half-lives: e.g., FVII has the shortest half-life (4–6 hours).

The coagulation cascade can be interpreted on the basis of the following tests:

- Partial thromboplastin time (PTT) measures the "intrinsic pathway." As such, it is affected by deficiencies in any of the following: prekallikrein, high-molecular weight kininogen, factors XII, XI, IX, VIII, X, V, II (prothrombin), and fibrinogen.
- International normalized ratio (INR) measures activity of factors VII, X, V, II, and fibrinogen.

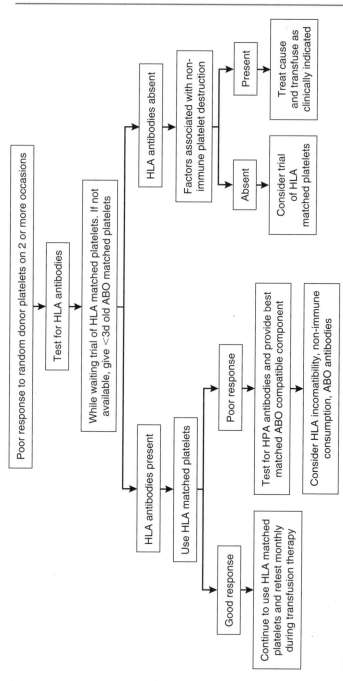

Figure 6-1 Management of platelet transfusion refractoriness.

Adaptation from the Clinical Policies Group. Guidelines for the Management of Platelet Transfusion Refractoriness.
http://hospital.blood.co.uk/library/pdf/guidePL.pdf May 2002.

Table 6-1   Interpretation of bleeding disorders according to PTT and INR.

		PTT	
		Increased	**Normal**
INR	**Increased**	FV, X, II or fibrinogen deficiency Liver failure Vitamin K deficiency DIC	FVII deficiency
	Normal	FVIII, IX, XI, XII deficiency Anti-phospholipid antibody Heparin contamination	FXIII deficiency Platelet disorders

Approach to the Bleeding Patient

- If patient is receiving heparin, discontinue heparin immediately.
- STAT blood work: CBC, blood smear, INR/PTT, fibrinogen, D-dimer; also consider liver enzymes, albumin, urea, creatinine.
- For low platelet count, transfuse 5–10 ml/kg to a maximum of 300 ml of platelets immediately (see section on transfuse platelet concentrates).
- For DIC: low platelets, low fibrinogen, high D-dimer, prolonged INR/PTT → transfuse fresh-frozen plasma (FFP): 10 ml/kg, cryoprecipitate: 1 U/kg and platelets 5–10 ml/kg.
- For prolonged INR and/or PTT: Immediately transfuse FFP 10 ml/kg (see section on transfuse frozen plasma [FP]) +/− vitamin K (phytonadione): 5 mg/dose IV over 10–20 minutes; watch for allergic reactions to IV vitamin K.
- For low hemoglobin: Transfuse 10 ml/kg of packed red blood cells (see section on transfuse packed red blood cells [PRBCs]).

- For life-threatening hemorrhage not responsive to platelets/FFP/cryoprecipitate, consider recombinant FVII (rFVIIa). Consult with hematologist experienced in use of rFVIIa.

Approach to the Nonbleeding Patient with Thrombocytopenia

See section on transfuse platelet concentrates.

Approach to the Nonbleeding Patient with Coagulopathy

- CBC, diff, blood smear, INR/PTT, fibrinogen, D-dimer; also consider liver enzymes, albumin, urea, creatinine and factor levels.
- For vitamin K deficiency, administer vitamin K at 2.5 to 5 mg/dose PO daily for 1–7 days, or 1–2 mg/dose IV daily for 1–7 days, titrating dose and length of treatment to effect; may also add vitamin K into TPN.
- Keep platelets $> 20 \times 10^9/l$.
- Minimize high-risk activities (e.g., contact sports).
- Correct coagulopathy prior to invasive procedures, such as lumbar punctures, surgeries, and central venous line insertions.

Transfusion Therapy Guidelines

- Children with cancer are often neutropenic, anemic, and/or thrombocytopenic secondary to chemotherapy, radiotherapy, or bone marrow infiltration (leukemia, neuroblastoma).
- Blood product transfusions are recommended when the risk of bleeding is high.

- Rather than transfusing on the basis of low hemoglobin or low platelet count, consider: (1) the patient's clinical status, such as presence of tachycardia, gallop rhythm, excessive fatigue or bleeding; (2) the mechanism of the patient's cytopenia; and (3) whether spontaneous improvement in the cytopenia (such as bone marrow recovery) is expected shortly.

Transfuse Packed Red Blood Cells (PRBCs)

- In bleeding state: Acute blood loss with symptoms and signs of hypovolemia not responsive to crystalloid or colloid infusions.
- In nonbleeding state:
  - Hb < 130 g/l: Patients with severe pulmonary disease.
  - Hb < 70 g/l: Patients receiving chemotherapy and/or radiotherapy.
- In operative setting:
  - Significant preoperative anemia (Hb < 80 g/l) in emergency surgical cases or in nonemergency cases where an alternate, effective therapy for anemia (e.g., iron therapy in a child with iron deficiency anemia) is not available.
  - Intraoperative blood loss > 15% of total blood volume.
  - Postoperative Hb < 80 g/l with symptoms and signs of anemia and where no alternate, effective therapy for anemia (e.g., iron therapy in a child with iron deficiency anemia) is available.
  - Avoid PRBC transfusion in leukemic children presenting with hyperleukocytosis (WBC > 100×10^9/l) and severe anemia, as it may cause increased viscosity and stroke, unless the patient is in congestive heart failure; in these cases transfuse very slowly (over 4 hours) with only 5 ml/kg of PRBC.

Transfuse Platelet Concentrates

- In bleeding state:
  - Platelet count (PC) $< 50 \times 10^9$/l with active bleeding.
  - PC $< 100 \times 10^9$/l with CNS bleeding.
- In nonbleeding state:
  - PC $< 10 \times 10^9$/l in a stable nonbleeding patient, without risk factors for hemorrhage (e.g., temperature $> 38.5°$C, coagulopathy, GI tract ulceration) and failure of platelet production.
  - PC $< 20 \times 10^9$/l in a stable nonbleeding patient, with risk factors for hemorrhage (e.g., temperature $> 38.5°$C, coagulopathy, GI tract ulceration, brain tumors, acute promyelocytic leukemia [APL]) and failure of platelet production.
  - PC $< 30 \times 10^9$/l in neonate with failure of platelet production.
- In operative setting:
  - PC $< 50 \times 10^9$/l with need for an invasive procedure in a patient with failure of platelet production.
  - PC $< 100 \times 10^9$/l and CNS surgery, or the need for an invasive procedure in a patient with a clinically significant coagulation abnormality, such as DIC.

Patients with HLA antibodies who are refractory to platelet transfusions may need HLA-matched single donor (apheresis) platelets.

Note: Platelet products supplied by Transfusion Services may be random donor platelets (RDP) (50–60 ml), buffy coat pool (300 ml), or single donor apheresis platelets (SDP) (300 ml). One buffy coat pool (from four donors) has same platelet content as five RDPs or one SDP.

Platelet dose for children is 5–10 ml/kg to a maximum of 300 ml (adult dose) per transfusion.

Transfuse Frozen Plasma (FP)

- In bleeding state:
  - Bleeding in a patient with documented coagulation factor deficiency and for whom specific factor concentrate is not available or effective.
  - Bleeding in a patient with a significantly prolonged INR or PTT ($>$ 1.5 $\times$ normal value/age) and for whom specific factor concentrate/alternate medical therapy (e.g., vitamin K) is not available or effective.
  - Bleeding during massive transfusion (in excess of 1 blood volume in less than 24 hours) not due to dilutional thrombocytopenia.
- In nonbleeding state: Reversal of warfarin in an emergency situation, such as before an invasive procedure with active bleeding.
- In operative setting:
  - Invasive procedure in a patient with documented coagulation factor deficiency and for whom specific factor concentrate is not available or effective.
  - Invasive procedure in a patient with a significantly prolonged INR or PTT ($>$ 1.5 $\times$ normal value/age) and for whom specific factor concentrate/alternate medical therapy (e.g., vitamin K) is not available or effective.

Note: Frozen plasma (FP, frozen within 24 hours) is used interchangeably with fresh-frozen plasma (FFP, frozen within 8 hours) for most clinical purposes.

Transfuse Cryoprecipitate

- In bleeding state:
  - Bleeding in patient with hypofibrinogenemia (fibrinogen levels $<$ 1.0 g/l) or dysfibrinogenemia (significantly

abnormal thrombin time not caused by heparin contamination; or significantly abnormal reptilase time).

○ Bleeding in patient with factor XIII deficiency (*when FXIII concentrate not available*).

- In nonbleeding state: No indication.
- In operative setting:
  ○ An invasive procedure in patient with hypofibrinogenemia or dysfibrinogenemia.
  ○ An invasive procedure in patient with factor XIII deficiency (*when FXIII concentrate is not available*).

Transfuse Albumin

- For acute correction of hypoalbuminemia *when clinically indicated.*
- For correction of hypovolemia *when colloid infusion is indicated.*
- For replacement therapy in phlebotomy or plasma exchange procedures use 5% albumin (or 25% albumin if concern about volume overload), give 0.5–1 g/kg to a maximum of 6 g/kg/day. Give over 2–4 hours. Consider giving 0.5–1 mg/kg of furosemide half way through infusion if trying to remove fluid.

Criteria for Transfusion of Cytomegalovirus Antibody Negative (Anti-CMV-Negative) Cellular Blood Products (RBCs and Platelets)

- CMV-seronegative bone marrow transplant recipients.
- CMV-seronegative patients who are likely candidates for bone marrow transplant (e.g., severe combined immunodeficiency, aplastic anemia).

- CMV-seronegative patients receiving *high-dose* chemotherapy for hematologic malignancies (e.g., leukemia, lymphoma) or malignant solid tumors (e.g., neuroblastoma, medulloblastoma).
- CMV-seronegative solid organ transplant recipients from CMV seronegative solid organ donors.
- CMV-seronegative patients infected with the human immunodeficiency (HIV) virus.
- CMV-seronegative pregnant females.
  - CMV seronegative means CMV IgG antibody negative.
  - All blood products in Canada are now prestorage leuko-reduced and therefore (as CMV is transmitted through leukocytes) considered to be at very low risk for transmitting CMV.
  - CMV-seronegative blood products should not be ordered for CMV-seropositive patients.

Criteria for Transfusion of Irradiated Cellular Blood Products (RBCs and Platelets)

The following patients must receive irradiated cellular blood products:

- Bone marrow transplant recipients.
- All patients on intensive chemotherapy protocols (hematologic malignancies and malignant solid tumors).
- Solid organ transplant recipients (heart, lung, small bowel transplants).
- Patients with congenital immunodeficiency disorders of cellular immunity such as severe combined immunodeficiency, DiGeorge syndrome, or deletion 22q syndrome.
- Premature infants and infants with known or suspected congenital or acquired immunodeficiency states.

Transfusion Reactions

Immediate Types

For any of the following types of transfusion reactions:

- Immediately stop transfusion.
- Run normal saline to keep vein open.
- Check all labels, forms, and patient identification.
- Inform blood transfusion laboratory.

Hemolytic

- Intravascular:
  - Etiology: Immune-mediated complement binding (e.g., ABO incompatibility).
- Extravascular:
  - Etiology: Immune-mediated noncomplement binding (e.g., Rh, Kelly, Duffy incompatibility).
  - Management: Keep well hydrated with IV normal saline to maintain urine output and prevent renal failure.

Fever/Chills

- Etiology:
  - HLA antibodies against donor leukocyte and platelet antigens.
  - Cytokine release from white cells during blood storage.
- Management:
  - Treat with acetaminophen; send blood cultures to rule out sepsis; do not restart transfusion.
  - For future transfusions, premedicate with acetaminophen; give leuko-reduced products if reactions recur despite premedication.

Note: All products in Canada are prestorage leuko-reduced. If severe reactions persist despite premedication and use of leuko-reduced products, consider washed red cells or plasma-reduced platelet concentrates.

Allergic

- Urticaria:
  - Etiology: Foreign antigens from donor plasma reacting with recipient IgE.
  - Management:
    - Treat with diphenhydramine 1–2 mg/kg/dose IV q 6 h (max 50 mg/dose).
    - May slowly restart blood transfusion in 15–30 minutes.
    - For next transfusion premedicate with diphenhydramine.
- Anaphylaxis:
  - Etiology: Antibody in recipient to donor plasma proteins (e.g., anti-IgA in recipient).
  - Management:
    - Treat with epinephrine 1:1000 (0.01 ml/kg IM; max 0.5 ml/dose) IM into the thigh; repeat after 5 minutes if needed.
    - Diphenhydramine (1–2 mg/kg/dose IV q 6 h to max of 50 mg/dose).
    - If wheezing give salbutamol 0.03 ml/kg in 3 ml NS by nebulizer (max of 1 ml/dose).
    - Consider hydrocortisone 5–10 mg/kg/dose IV q 6 h if severe.

Note: If severe allergic or anaphylactic reactions persist despite premedication, consider washed red cells or plasma-reduced platelet concentrates.

Hemorrhage

- Due to dilutional thrombocytopenia after massive transfusion: Transfuse platelets.

Transfusion-Related Acute Lung Injury (TRALI)

- Etiology: Passive transfer of leuko-agglutinating antibodies resulting in noncardiogenic pulmonary edema and resultant hypoxia. Usually occurs within 4 hours of transfusion.
- Management: Supportive.

Transfusion-Related Circulatory Overload

- Give furosemide 0.5–2 mg/kg/dose IV halfway through or immediately after transfusion.

Delayed Types

Hemolytic

- Etiology: Anamnestic immune response occurring 7–14 days after a transfusion. Occurs because antibodies in recipient are present in low levels, thus antibody screen is negative. Incompatible blood is then given, boosting the recipient's antibody production, resulting in delayed hemolysis.

Alloimmunization

- Etiology: Immune sensitization to donor red cell antigens.

Graft-vs.-Host Disease (GVHD)

- Etiology: Usually occurs 8–10 days after transfusion and is a result of functioning donor lymphocytes transfused into an immunocompromised, or HLA-similar immuno-competent, recipient.

- Presentation: Skin rash, diarrhea, liver dysfunction; can be fatal.

Posttransfusion Purpura

- Etiology: Platelet antibodies, usually against HPA-1a.

Platelet Refractoriness

- A platelet transfusion of 10 ml/kg is expected to raise the patient's platelet count by 30–60 $\times$ $10^9/l$.
- Poor response to platelet transfusion: Defined as the consistent inability to increase platelet count following transfusion.
- Immune refractoriness to platelets: Failure to obtain an increment in platelet counts of more than 10 $\times$ $10^9/l$ on two consecutive posttransfusion counts (measured 10 min to 1 hour after transfusion).
- Nonimmune platelet destruction/consumption: Decreased platelet survival as measured by a more rapid than expected fall in platelet count at 18–24 h post-transfusion.

Immune

- HLA alloantibodies.
- HPA alloantibodies.
- Platelet autoantibodies.
- ABO incompatibility.
- Drug-dependent platelet antibodies.
- Immune complexes.

Seen most often in patients who receive multiple platelet transfusions, and likelihood increases with increasing number of transfusions.

Nonimmune

- Infection and its treatment, particularly amphotericin-B.
- Splenomegaly.
- DIC.
- Bleeding.

References

American Association of Blood Banks. Summary of use of CMV safe blood. Bulletin #97-2, Table #3. Bethesda, MD: American Association of Blood Banks.

Bakdash S, Yazer M. What every physician should know about transfusion reactions. *CMAJ*. 2007;177(2): .

Blanchette VS, Hume HA, Levy GJ, Luban NLC, Strauss RG. Guidelines for auditing pediatric blood transfusion practices. *Am J Dis Child*. 1991;145: 787–796.

Blanchette V, Lau W, Carcao M. Canadian Blood Services Circular of Information. The Hospital for Sick Children; 2008.

British Committee for Standards in Haematology Transfusion Task Force: Writing Group. Transfusion guidelines for neonates and older children. *Brit J Haematol*. 2004;124:433–453.

Cheng A, Williams B, Sivarajan B. *HSC Handbook of Pediatrics* 10th ed. St. Louis: Elsevier; 2003.

Gaydos LA, Freireich EJ, Mantel N. The quantitative relation between platelet count and hemorrhage in patients with acute leukemia. *N Engl J Med*. 1962;266:905–909.

Gmür J, Burger J, Schanz U, Fehr J, Schaffner A. Safety of stringent prophylactic platelet transfusion policy for patients with acute leukaemia. *Lancet*. 1991;338:1223–1226.

Goodnough L, Brecher M, Kanter M, AuBuchon J. Transfusion medicine: first of two parts. *NEJM*. 1999;340(6):438–447.

Hillyer CD, Strauss RG, Luban NLC. *Handbook of Pediatric Transfusion Medicine*. Elsevier Academic Press; 2004.

Lau E, Drugs and Therapeutics Committee. *SickKids Drug Handbook and Formulary*. Toronto, ON; 2007–2008.

Pediatric Transfusion: A Physician's Handbook. 2nd ed. Bethesda, MD: AABB Press; 2006.

Platelet transfusion for patients with cancer: clinical practice guidelines of the American Society of Clinical Oncology. *J Clin Oncol*. 2001;19:1519–1538.

Roseff SD, Luban NL, Manno CS. Guidelines for assessing appropriateness of pediatric transfusion. *Transfusion*. 2002:42:1398–1413.

Hyperleukocytosis/ Hyperviscosity Syndrome

Angela Punnett and Oussama Abla

Outline

- Introduction
- Precautions
- Clinical Presentation
- Initial Management
- Leukapheresis

Introduction

- Hyperleukocytosis is defined as a presenting white blood cell count (WBC) $> 100 \times 10^9$/l.
- Seen in acute leukemias (AML > ALL) and CML.
- May be symptomatic or asymptomatic.

- Symptoms due primarily to increased blood viscosity and leukostasis (sludging of circulating leukemic blasts in the microvasculature).
- Leukostasis is more common in AML; myeloblasts are larger and more adherent than lymphoblasts.

Precautions

- Increased incidence in infants, AML-M4/M5 subtypes, ALL-T cell and precursor B-cell with poor risk genetics (e.g., Philadelphia chromosome-positive and MLL-gene rearrangement).
- Packed red blood cell (PRBC) transfusions lead to increased blood viscosity and have been associated with increased risk of death.

Clinical Presentation

- Leukostasis primarily affects the central nervous system (CNS), the lungs, and the kidneys.
- Most early deaths are due to respiratory failure and/or intracranial hemorrhage.
- CNS presentations: Headache, confusion, somnolence, stupor, coma, dizziness, gait instability, blurred vision, papilledema, and cranial nerve defects.
- Pulmonary presentations: Exertional dyspnea, hypoxemia, severe respiratory distress:
  - CXR may be normal or with nonspecific diffuse infiltrates.
- Other symptoms include:
  - Vascular: Retinal vein thrombosis, retinal hemorrhage, myocardial infarction, limb ischemia, bowel infarctions, priapism, renal vein thrombosis.
  - Fever.

○ Thrombocytopenia, DIC.

○ Renal failure secondary to severe tumor lysis.

Initial Management

- Correct thrombocytopenia/DIC:
  - ○ *Always* perform a manual platelet count (more accurate).
  - ○ Transfuse platelets/FFP as needed (no significant effect on viscosity).
- Avoid PRBC transfusions or transfuse minimal amounts of PRBCs (3–5 cc/kg, very slowly) in symptomatic patients (e.g. congestive heart failure).
- Prevent and treat tumor lysis syndrome:
  - ○ Rasburicase for hyperuricemia (see Chapter 16).
- Leukocyto-reduction:
  - ○ Early start of chemotherapy most important.
  - ○ Hydroxyurea for CML patients.
  - ○ Leukapheresis.

Leukapheresis

- Separation and removal of excessive mononuclear cells from the blood.
- Controversial benefit or lack of harm in existing literature.
- Indications:
  - ○ Individualized approach.
  - ○ Consider for ALL/AML with WBC $> 100 \times 10^9/l$ and symptomatic (e.g., CNS or pulmonary leukostasis).
  - ○ Consider for asymptomatic patients with ALL and WBC $> 400 \times 10^9/l$.
  - ○ Consider for asymptomatic patients with AML and WBC $> 200 \times 10^9/l$.

- Contraindications: Patients with acute promyelocytic leukemia (AML-M3) as it may cause catastrophic bleeding.
- Clinical notes:
  - Notify ICU, blood bank, and apheresis team early.
  - Double blood volume leukapheresis reduces initial WBC by almost 50 %.
    - Volume calculated as [TBV × wt (kg) × 2].
    - TBV (total blood volume) = neonates 100 ml/kg, infants and small children 80 ml/kg, older children 70 ml/kg.
  - Prime circuit using reconstituted whole blood (FFP and PRBCs) with Hct as close as possible to the patient's Hct.
  - Use CMV-negative, irradiated blood products.
  - Maintain isovolemia:
    - May return prime to patient if weight > 20 kg.
    - Other replacement fluids: FFP/platelets (preferred), 5 % albumin.
- Complications:
  - Fluid shifts/hypotension, hypertension.
  - Electrolyte abnormalities: Hypocalcemia, hypomagnesemia, and hypokalemia:
    - Check CBC, diff, ionized Ca, K, Mg, Phosphate, albumin within 2 hours pre- and 30 minutes post-procedure.
    - Citrate is used as anticoagulant during leukapheresis:
      - Effect on ionized calcium level and on magnesium, potassium, pH and bicarbonate levels.
      - IV Ca gluconate infusion is used to avoid citrate toxicity. Beware of IV Ca infusions in presence of hyperphosphatemia → may cause nephrocalcinosis.

- Temperature fluctuations.
- Arrhythmias: bradycardia.
- Line-related femoral vein thrombosis.
- Anemia, thrombocytopenia.
- Coagulopathy.
- Hypoalbuminemia, edema.
- Respiratory and cardiac compromise.
- Chills related to citrate.
- Allergic reactions to blood products.

Follow-Up

- Patient WBC following leukapheresis is not always a good indicator of efficiency of the procedure due to possible recruitment of sequestered cells.
- Patients may develop a systemic inflammatory response syndrome (SIRS) following leukapheresis and the initiation of chemotherapy.
- → the use of steroids in SIRS may be beneficial.

Tip

- The use of leukapheresis must not delay the timely initiation of chemotherapy as the latter is the primary goal of management.

References

Kim HC. Therapeutic pediatric apheresis. *J Clin Apheresis*. 2000;15:129–157.

Lowe EJ, Pui CH, Hancock ML, et al. Early complications in children with ALL presenting with hyperleukocytosis. *Pediatr. Blood Cancer*. 2005;45:10–15.

Majhail NS, Lichtin A. Acute leukemia with a very high leukocyte count: confronting a medical emergency. *Cleveland Clinic J Med.* 2004;71:633–637.

Smith JW, Weinstein R, & Hillyer KL for the AABB Hemapheresis Committee. Therapeutic apheresis: A summary of current indication categories endorsed by the AABB and the American Society for Apheresis. *Transfusion.* 2003;43:820–822.

c h a p t e r   8

Infectious Complications in Pediatric Cancer Patients

Amy Lee Chong, Elyse Zelunka, and Lillian Sung

Outline

- Introduction
- Management of Fever in Oncology Patients
- Postoperative Fevers in Oncology Patients
- Herpes and Varicella Infections
- *Pneumocystis jirveci* Infection

Introduction

- Children with malignancies or those posthematopoietic stem cell transplant (HSCT) are at increased risk of infection-related morbidity and mortality.
- Risk factors include leukopenia, skin and mucosal defects, malnutrition, diminished antibody responses

associated with the underlying disease, and immuno-supressant/antineoplastic treatments.

- Patients are at risk for common community-acquired infections and from organisms colonizing their skin and gastrointestinal tract (e.g., Coagulase-negative *Staphylococci, Staphylococcus aureus*, *Escherichia coli*, and *Klebsiella* species).

- Empiric antibiotic, antifungal, or antiviral therapies are important interventions particularly in the setting of fever in neutropenic patients or in any oncology patient who appears clinically unwell as host response to infection is often severely depressed.

Risk Factors for Significant Infections

- All children with fever and neutropenia (absolute neutrophil count or ANC $< 0.5 \times 10^9$/l) receiving antineoplastic agents.

- All children receiving antineoplastic agents who have indwelling catheters, irrespective of white blood cell count (WBC).

- All children who are within 6 months of HSCT, irrespective of WBC or whether they are receiving immunosuppressive agents at presentation.

- All immunocompromised children who present clinically unwell, irrespective of treatment status, fever, or WBC.

- All immunocompromised children who develop fever following a major surgical procedure.

Definition of Neutropenia

- Chemotherapy-induced neutropenia is defined as a low neutrophil count ($< 2 \times 10^9$/l) and can be graded as per the common toxicity criteria of the National Cancer Institute as follows:

- ○ Grade 1 : ANC $\geq$ 1.5 to $<$ 2 $\times$ 10^9/l.
- ○ Grade 2 : ANC $\geq$ 1.0 to $<$ 1.5 $\times$ 10^9/l.
- ○ Grade 3 : ANC $\geq$ 0.5 to $<$ 1.0 $\times$ 10^9/l.
- ○ Grade 4 : ANC $\leq$ 0.5 $\times$ 10^9/l.
- As the ANC decreases, the risk of infection increases, with the greatest risk being at counts less than $<$ 0.5 $\times$ 10^9/l.
- The longer the duration of neutropenia (typical period is 7 days following chemotherapy with evidence of recovery thereafter), the greater the risk of infection-related morbidity and mortality.

Common Presenting Symptoms of Infection

- Fever can be defined as a single oral temperature of $\geq$ 38.3°C (101°F) or a temperature of $\geq$ 38.0°C (100.4°F) for $\geq$ 1 h as per the Infectious Disease Society of America Fever and Neutropenia Guidelines Panel. However, controversy exists as to the accepted values, and the exact temperatures used to define fever vary in each institution.
- Fever is often the earliest clinical sign of infection and should result in prompt clinical assessment of the child for a possible focus.
- Many patients have no symptoms other than fever +/− constitutional symptoms.
- Absence of a fever is not an indication to withhold antibiotic therapy in patients who have localizing signs of possible infection or who appear unwell.
- Clinical signs such as respiratory compromise, a tender abdomen, or a red/tender central venous line (CVL) site may indicate a source of an infection.

- Exercise caution with patients receiving corticosteroids, as they may present with an infection but in the absence of a fever.

Antibiotic Prophylaxis

- *Pneumocystis jirovecii* pneumonia (PJP, previously called PCP) prophylaxis is indicated for children with severe lymphopenia including all children with leukemia, those undergoing HSCT, and some children with brain and solid tumors (refer to later section on PCP prophylaxis guidelines).
- The use of other prophylactic antibiotics is controversial.
- Some antineoplastic regimens associated with severe lymphopenia recommend fungal and viral prophylaxis (with medications such as fluconazole and acyclovir) as part of their treatment protocols.
- At the Hospital for Sick Children, routine antibacterial prophylaxis is not used; however, the use of antifungal and/or antiviral prophylaxis may be included in some treatment protocols.
- Prophylactic medications should be continued during the empiric treatment of fever unless the presenting illness precludes their administration or requires different doses to be administered.
- In a patient with documented prolonged neutropenia, the discontinuation of cotrimoxazole (for PCP prophylaxis) in view of a possible contributing effect should be considered. If cotrimoxazole is discontinued, alternate agents must be initiated for PCP prophylaxis until neutropenia resolves.

Management of Infection in Oncology Patients

Do all Febrile Children Need to Be Admitted?

- Not all children who are seen in the emergency department for assessment of a fever require admission.
- Any child who is clinically well or has an obvious focus of a localised infection (e.g., otitis media, tonsillitis, UTI), can be considered for discharge, provided they have an ANC $> 0.5 \times 10^9$/l.
- Cultures should be taken from peripheral and central venous sites, as well as any sites of possible infection before discharge; consider giving a prescription for oral antibiotics to treat focal infection, if present; alert the patient's primary oncologist for further follow-up.
- Some investigators have proposed home management on oral/parenteral antibiotic therapy, empirically, for a very select group of clinically well patients who have ANC $< 0.5 \times 10^9$/l. This is not the current policy at the Hospital for Sick Children.

Investigations at Presentation

- CBC/differential.
- Serum electrolytes and creatinine: Modify antibiotic doses if evidence of renal compromise.
- Aerobic blood cultures (peripheral vein and each lumen of central lines): Ensure that adequate volumes are obtained for more reliable results, which is dependent on the age/weight of the child.
- Anaerobic blood cultures should be obtained if infection of the gastrointestinal tract (e.g., typhilitis) or an abscess of the head, neck, or mediastinum is suspected.

Consider If Clinically Indicated

- Urine (if dipstix positive or clinical symptoms) and stool cultures.
- Swabs of any sites of possible infection.
- Nasopharyngeal aspirate for respiratory viruses +/− *Mycoplasma*, *Bordetella*.
- Viral scrapings of any vesicular lesions (contact a virologist if available).
- Radiological investigations (X-ray/ultrasound/CT) as indicated by presenting symptoms.
- Review prior microbiology results for multiresistant micro-organisms (e.g., MRSA) and for prior viral infections (e.g., HSV/EBV/CMV).
- If a patient has been transferred from another institution, MRSA swabs will be required.
- Note: Acquisition of blood cultures (peripheral vein and central venous catheter) are essential to the investigation of every febrile patient. Other specimens if clinically indicated (urine, secretions, and stool) are preferred but should not cause an untimely delay in starting appropriate empiric therapy.

Initial Empiric Antibiotic Choice*

- The decision as to which antibiotics to start in an admitted oncology patient relates to the clinical status of the patient (i.e., stable versus unstable) at presentation, the patient's drug allergy history, and on the clinical findings that may suggest a possible focus of infection.
- Initial antibiotic coverage should be broad spectrum, including those which offer appropriate coverage for most

* For drug dosage please see Chapter 19.

commonly seen gram-positive and gram-negative micro-organisms (as per local bacterial isolates and resistance profiles).

- The Hospital for Sick Children currently recommends that the *stable patient:* is treated with tazobactam + piperacilllin (e.g., Tazocin) and gentamicin *or* ciprofloxacin and gentamicin and clindamycin in those with a severe beta-lactam allergy. The addition of vancomycin should be considered if there is clinical evidence of a possible CVL infection, such as discharge, a red tender site, and/or tracking over the line.
- In an *unstable patient* who presents in septic shock with hemodynamic instability, second-line antibiotics should be started immediately; these include meropenem and vancomycin and gentamicin *or* ciprofloxacin and amikacin and vancomycin in those with a severe beta-lactam allergy.
- Consult local institutional policy on the management of fever/neutropenia to confirm the recommended empiric antibiotic choices. In addition, drug choice and/or doses should be modified where there is evidence of renal compromise and aminoglycosides should be avoided in patients with significant pre-existing hearing loss.

Important Points

- Central cultures should be taken daily while patient remains febrile. Peripheral cultures are not recommended in patients already receiving broad-spectrum antibiotic therapy.
- All antibiotics should be administered via CVLs and alternated if there is more than one lumen.
- CBC with differential and renal profile should be monitored for count recovery and for possible renal toxicity while on antibiotic therapy.

- Aminoglycosides and vancomycin plasma concentrations should be closely monitored and drug doses adjusted accordingly.
- On identification of a positive culture, repeat cultures should be taken. An antibiotic directed specifically at the isolated organism should be added to the empiric broad-spectrum coverage if the empiric antibiotics are not adequate.
- Criteria for CVL removal:
    - Positive blood cultures for *Candida sp., Staphylococcus aureus.*
    - Evidence of a tunnel infection.
    - Persistent positive blood cultures.
    - Clinical deterioration with known positive blood cultures.
- Evidence of a possible superficial mucosal fungal infection should be treated with oral fluconazole. Remember to evaluate the patient's current or planned drug regimen for possible interactions with fluconazole.
- Identification of a *Staphylococcus aureus* infection should prompt consideration of an echocardiogram to rule out endocarditis and, if clinically indicated, a bone scan to rule out osteomyelitis.

Supportive Care

- Vital signs should be assessed q 4 h, unless clinical presentation indicates a more frequent regimen.
- Acetaminophen can be administered for fever control, provided initial cultures have been taken. A baseline temperature should be recorded before each dose of acetaminophen, to allow for accurate assessment of fever over any 24-hour period. At the Hospital for Sick Children the use of ibuprofen as an antipyretic is not recommended in oncology patients.

- For pain relief, narcotics such as oral codeine or oral/IV morphine are useful first-line agents. Avoid giving acetaminophen for pain as it may mask a fever.
- All antineoplastic agents should be held, in consultation with the responsible oncologist.
- In patients who are neutropenic following HSCT and who are hemodynamically unstable at presentation or deteriorating, granulocyte-colony-stimulating-factor or G-CSF (Filgrastim at 5 mcg/kg/dose IV) should be initiated.
- In non-HSCT neutropenic patients who are hemodynamically unstable at presentation, clinically deteriorate, have a positive blood culture, or have findings suggestive of an invasive fungal infection on imaging, the use of G-CSF should be considered.

The Deteriorating Patient*

- If a previously stable patient should clinically deteriorate or become hemodynamically unstable while receiving first-line antibiotics → coverage should be modified to meropenem and vancomycin and amikacin *or* ciprofloxacin and amikacin and vancomycin in those with a beta-lactam allergy. The responsible oncologist should be informed, and an infectious diseases consult should be requested.

Discontinuation of Antibiotics

- Patients are considered to be at high risk of bacteremia if they are:
  - Receiving induction therapy for a malignancy known to significantly involve the bone marrow (e.g., AML,

---

* For drug dosage please see Chapter 19.

relapsed ALL, stage III/IV Burkitt's or large B cell lymphoma).

○ Or receiving antineoplastic protocols known to be associated with a high risk of infectious morbidity/ mortality.

○ Or undergoing autologous or allogeneic HSCT.

• Fever in such patients should be managed conservatively, and decisions to discontinue broad-spectrum antibiotics after 7 to 14 days of therapy regardless of ANC should be individualized.

General Guidelines

• Antibiotics can be discontinued in a stable patient who has negative cultures after 48 hours of antibiotic therapy, has been afebrile for > 24 hours, and is showing evidence of count recovery (ANC, monocytes, or platelets).

• Consider stopping antibiotics regardless of ANC if patient is not in the aforementioned group of at risk patients, has evidence of count recovery (increased ANC, monocytes, or platelets), and meets the following criteria:

○ Did not present with clinical sepsis or hemodynamic instability.

○ Fever did not persist beyond 96 hours.

○ Is clinically well and not in need of any other inpatient care.

○ A follow-up plan with primary team has been arranged.

• It is not necessary to keep the patient in hospital for 24 hours following discontinuation of IV antibiotic therapy.

• Any recurrence of fever should be approached as a *de novo fever* in an immunocompromised host and requires immediate evaluation (see prolonged fever section below).

- A patient who presented with cardiovascular instability, or one who deteriorates clinically while on treatment, should receive a minimum of 7–10 days of IV antibiotics. Discontinuation of antibiotics should be decided on an individual basis.

- Long-term use of broad-spectrum antibiotics is associated with increasing risk of fungal infection, and this risk should be considered in the treatment of patients with prolonged fever or neutropenia.

Prolonged Fever

- When a fever persists for > 5 to 7 days, or recurs after > 5 to 7 days of antibiotic administration after a period of defervesence, investigation for invasive fungal infection should be performed (blood and urine cultures, CT chest [+/− sinuses depending on the age of the child], U/S abdomen, and swabs of any possible sites) and empiric antifungal therapy started. The scheduling of imaging should not delay antifungal administration.

Empiric Antifungal Therapy*

- Fungal infections such as *Candida* and *Aspergillus* are a common cause of secondary and, less frequently, primary infection in patients who have received broad-spectrum antibiotics, prolonged steroid therapy, and/or who have skin/mucosal defects or indwelling catheters.

* For drug dosage please see Chapter 19.

- The choice of empiric antifungal is made on the basis of patient age and risk factors for actual fungal infection. Institutional policies should be consulted for up-to-date information regarding the formulary empiric antifungal agents.

- Currently, we recommend that children less than 2 years of age should receive conventional amphotericin unless they have preexisting significant renal impairment or develop significant renal impairment while receiving conventional amphotericin. The latter children should receive liposomal amphotericin.

- Children 2 years of age and older who are at high risk of having an actual fungal infection when empiric antifungal agents are initiated should receive caspofungin.

- The decision to start empiric intravenous antifungal therapy using conventional amphotericin should be discussed with the staff oncologist. The infectious disease service should be consulted regarding suspected or proven fungal infection.

Important Points

- Children receiving amphotericin (conventional and lipid) can develop infusion-related reactions (fevers, chills, rigors, headache, nausea), hypokalemia, and nephrotoxicity.

- Premedication with acetaminophen and diphenhydramine is routinely given to prevent amphotericin-induced fevers and rigors. Meperidine may be given before amphotericin doses to prevent rigors and p.r.n. q 2 h during the amphotericin infusion to treat rigors.

- Premedication with hydrocortisone should be discussed with the staff oncologist prior to use. It is usually reserved for infusion-related reactions that cannot be managed with the aforementioned premedications, in patients who must continue to receive amphotericin rather than an alternate antifungal agent (caspofungin or an azole). Unless otherwise contraindicated, a normal saline load (10 ml/kg; max 1 liter) should be given intravenously prior to each amphotericin dose (conventional and lipid) to prevent amphotericin-induced nephrotoxicity.

- Premedications can usually be weaned with continued administration of amphotericin.

Discontinuation of Antifungal Agents

- Discontinuation of antifungal therapy ideally coincides with:
  - Resolution of fever.
  - Evidence of count recovery.
  - Absence of imaging indicative of presumed, probable, or actual fungal infection on initial fungal workup or its resolution, if evident on initial fungal workup.
- This decision should be made on a case-by-case basis after discussion with the staff oncologist.
- Treatment of presumed, probable, or actual fungal infection and use of oral antifungal agents (e.g., voriconazole and posaconazole) should be guided by the infectious diseases service.

Postoperative Fevers in Oncology Patients

- Surgical oncology patients who have received chemotherapy may require empiric antibiotic therapy even if they are not neutropenic as they have an underlying immunosuppressed state. Therefore, fevers in oncology patients who have undergone major surgery require an immediate and comprehensive assessment, which should include:

○ Physical exam.

○ CBC, differential.

○ Blood cultures (peripheral vein and central venous catheters).

○ Consultation of the oncology service.

- Consideration should be given to also obtain:

○ Urine culture (especially in those who have been catheterized during their surgery).

○ Wound, drain, other fluid cultures based on clinical status.

○ Chest X-ray.

- In a *clinically stable and nonneutropenic* surgical oncology patient, the decision to start an antibiotic is often at the physician's discretion. Many patients in the immediate postoperative period are already receiving antibiotic prophylaxis such as a cephalosporin as part of postoperative management, and continuation of these antibiotics may be appropriate.

- If there is a potential infectious focus then antibiotic coverage should be modified as indicated.

- In the patient who is no longer receiving antibiotics, assessment and acquisition of cultures without initiating empiric antibiotics is also acceptable, provided no focus is identified and the patient is closely monitored.

- In the *clinically unstable and/or neutropenic* surgical oncology patient, an immediate assessment is required, cultures should be taken, and empiric antibiotics commenced (as per initial empiric antibiotic choice above), or existing antibiotics modified to broad-spectrum coverage.

Herpes and Varicella Infections

Presentation and Management

- The presence of any vesicular lesion(s) in a child with a malignancy should be treated as possible herpes or varicella infection until proven otherwise.

- A scraping of the lesion(s) should be sent for PCR and acyclovir should be started immediately.

- In all children, blood for herpes/varicella PCR, liver enzymes, and amylase should be checked. Rule out hepatitis or pancreatitis suggestive of disseminated infection.

- Disseminated cases should be admitted to an isolation room in an infectious disease ward. Patients presenting with Herpes zoster of one dermatome only, can be admitted to the hematology/oncology unit using appropriate isolation procedures.

- Isolated oral herpes lesions can be treated initially with a course of oral acyclovir, provided the patient is not receiving a severely immunocompromising regimen and there is close follow-up of the lesions arranged.

- If the patient is unable to tolerate oral dosing, or there is a suspicion of more extensive herpes infection or presentation of rash suggestive of varicella, then the the patient should be admitted to receive intravenous acyclovir.

- Bacterial cultures should also be obtained and empiric antibiotics (see above) should be started if a neutropenic patient develops fever while being treated with antiviral agents.

Varicella Exposure

- Any child with no evidence of prior varicella immunity who comes into potential contact with a varicella infected child should receive VZIG (125 units/10 kg IM) as soon as possible, up to a maximum of 96 h post-exposure.

- Parents should be informed that their child may still develop varicella, the first onset of rash being 10 days from exposure, and will remain at risk until 28 days post, due to the administration of the VZIG.

Pneumocystis jirovecii Infection

Etiology

- *Pneumocystic jirovecii* is the organism that is responsible for human pneumocystis pneumoniae (PCP).
- Originally classified as a protozoan, pneumocystis is now referred to as a fungus.
- Most individuals are infected by the age of 4 years; PCP is thought to occur by either reactivation of a latent infection or aerosol transmission.
- Main risk factors: children with deficiencies in cellular immunity and those receiving corticosteroids.
- Risk of development of PCP in this group = 5–15% with a mortality rate of 20–30%.

Clinical Presentation

- Relative rapid onset (over a few days) of hypoxia that may be accompanied by nonproductive cough.
- Hypoxemia secondary to PCP produces a characteristic wide alveolar-arterial oxygen gradient.
- Physical examination: Tachypnea, tachycardia, and normal findings on lung auscultation.

- Chest X-ray maybe normal despite the hypoxemia; diffuse, fine, ground-glass interstitial infiltrates are common.
- Other atypical radiographic features are small effusions, focal consolidation, small nodules or cavities, pneumatoceles, and lymphadenopathy.
- CT scan: Diffuse interstitial and nodular parenchymal involvement, even if chest X-ray results are normal.
- Nuclear medicine imaging is not recommended; results are nonspecific.

Diagnosis

- Organism burden is lower in non-AIDS patients, making noninvasive diagnosis difficult.
- A forced sputum sample should be considered; however, it only has a diagnostic yield of 30–55 % and therefore is rarely useful for the diagnosis of PCP.
- Bronchoscopy with a bronchoalveolar lavage (BAL) should be performed in all patients with negative sputum results.
- Transbronchial biopsies further increase the diagnostic yield to over 90 %.

Treatment*

- Cotrimoxazole is the drug of choice for treatment of PCP.
- Corticosteroids appear to be beneficial as an adjunct to cotrimoxazole in the treatment of HIV-infected adults with moderate to severe PCP; however, no controlled studies in children have been done.

* For drug dosage please see Chapter 19.

- Most experts would include corticosteroids as part of therapy for children with moderate to severe PCP disease. The optimal dose and duration of corticosteroid therapy for children have not been determined.

Prophylaxis *

- Patients should receive PCP prophylaxis if they are:
  - Undergoing treatment for ALL or AML.
  - Undergoing treatment for a malignancy where corticosteroids are used in moderate to high doses for periods longer than 4 weeks.
  - Have received a blood or bone marrow transplant.
  - Have severe combined immunodeficiency.
- Prophylactic therapy for haematology/oncology patients may be discontinued 3–6 months postcompletion of their chemotherapy protocol.
- Prophylactic therapy for blood or bone marrow transplant patients should be given from engraftment until 6 months post-HSCT and beyond 6 months in patients with GVHD on continued immunosuppression.
- Cotrimoxazole is the gold standard of prophylaxis.
- If a patient develops neutropenia or mild rash while receiving cotrimoxazole, hold dose for 2 weeks and rechallenge.
- Aerosolized pentamidine, dapsone, and atovaquone are alternates if rechallenge with cotrimoxazole fails.
- Cotrimoxazole should not be given to post-HSCT patients who are still platelet-transfusion dependent (platelets must be $> 50 \times 10^9$/L to begin therapy) as it may worsen thrombocytopenia.

* For drug dosage please see Chapter 19.

References

American Academy of Pediatrics. *Pneumocystis jirovecii* Infections. In: Pickering LK, ed. *Red Book: 2006 Report of the Committee on Infectious Diseases*. 27th ed. Elk Gove Village, IL: American Academy of Pediatrics; 2006: [500–504].

Gafter-Gvili A, Fraser A, Paul M, et al. Antibiotic prophylaxis for bacterial infections in afebrile neutropenic patients following chemotherapy. *Cochrane Database Syst Rev*. 2005;(4):CD004386.

Hughes WT, Armstrong D, Bodey GP, et al. 2002 guidelines for the use of antimicrobial agents in neutropenic patients with cancer. *Clin Infect Dis*. 2002;34(6):730–751.

Hughes WT, Rivera GK, Schell MJ , et al. Successful intermittent chemoprophylaxis for *Pneumocystis carinii* pneumonitis. *N Eng J Med*. 1987;316: 1627–1632.

Koh AY, Alexander S, Pizzo PA. Infections in children with cancer. In: Long SS, Pickering LK, Prober CG, eds. *Principals and Practice of Pediatric Infectious Diseases*. 2nd ed. Philadelphia, PA: Churchill Livingstone; 2002:575–582

Pui CH, Hughtes WT, Evans WE, et al. Prevention of *Pneumocystis carinii* pneumonia in children with cancer [Letter]. *J Clin Oncol*. 1994;12: 1522–1525.

Rodriguez M, Fishman JA. Prevention of infection due to *Pneumocystis* spp. in human immunodeficiency virus-negative immunocompromised patients. *Clin Microbiol Rev*. 2004;17:770–782.

Walsh TJ, Roilides E, Groll AH, et al. Infectious complications in pediatric cancer patients. In: Pizzo PA, Poplack DG, eds. *Principals and Practice of Pediatric Oncology*. 5th ed. Philadelphia, PA: Lippincott Williams & Wilkins; 2005:1269–1329

c h a p t e r   9

Menses Suppression

Angela Punnett and Tracey Taylor

Outline

- Etiology
- Precautions
- Clinical Presentation
- Initial Management
- Follow-Up
- Tips

Etiology

- Severe thrombocytopenia following myelosuppressive chemotherapy may be associated with menorrhagia in postpubertal girls.
- Abdominal-pelvic radiation and/or alkylating agents given to postpubertal girls can predispose to premature ovarian failure later in life.

- No convincing evidence that any pharmacologic intervention mitigates or prevents premature ovarian failure under these circumstances.

Precautions

- Discuss contraceptive methods and safe sexual practices with all sexually active patients, and counsel them regarding teratogenic potential of chemotherapy as well as infectious risks of intercourse.
- Gynecology (GYN) referral is recommended for patients who:
  - ○ Have uncontrolled menorrhagia with adequate platelet counts.
  - ○ Are about to undergo hematopoietic stem cell transplantation (HSCT).
  - ○ Seek contraception.
  - ○ Will require > 6 months of menses suppression.
- A method of contraception appropriate to the patients' lifestyle, underlying disease, and risk factors should be offered in consultation with GYN or adolescent medicine.
- Decreased contraceptive efficacy or increased breakthrough bleeding can occur if receiving rifampin, phenobarbital, carbamazepine, phenytoin, or antibiotics concurrently with oral contraceptives. A barrier method is recommended for contraception during such periods.

Clinical Presentation

- These guidelines are aimed at preventing menorrhagia during chemotherapy or HSCT.

Initial Management

- Patients who can tolerate IM injections and have no evidence of osteoporosis:
  - GnRH analog, Leuprolide 3.75 mg IM once monthly, or 11.25 mg IM every 3 months. Give the first dose on day 14 to 28 of the patient's menstrual cycle and monthly (if giving 3.75 mg), or every 3 months (if giving 11.25 mg), thereafter if continued menses suppression is required.
  - Side effects: hot flushes, blurred vision, dizziness, edema, redness and swelling at the injection site, nausea, paresthesias, insomnia, weight gain, breast tenderness, mood changes, vaginitis, cardiac arrhythmias, deepening of the voice, and increased hair growth.
  - It is important to educate patients that Leuprolide does not provide adequate contraception nor does it prevent sexually transmitted diseases during intercourse.
- To control breakthrough bleeding despite prophylaxis with leuprolide, give:
  - Ovral® 1 tablet (250 µg d-norgestrel and 50 µg ethinyl estradiol) once daily PO.
  - Ovral® tablets may be given per vagina at twice the oral dose. Consider this route if patient is unable to take PO (severe mucositis, nausea, or diarrhea) and the patient is not neutropenic.
  - When flow is stopped and a minimum of 14 days of therapy has been administered, discontinue Ovral®.
  - A small amount of bleeding may occur on discontinuation of Ovral®.

- For patients on oral contraceptives for menses suppression and/or contraception:
  - Discontinue at least 2 weeks prior to a planned surgery that will lead to a period of immobilization, or as soon as possible before emergency surgery.
  - Common side effects especially in first 3 months: spotting, dysmenorrhea, nausea, breast tenderness, sodium/fluid retention, or bloating. Less frequently: reduced glucose tolerance, headaches, vaginal candidiasis, photosensitivity, or changes in body/facial hair.
  - May rarely cause life-threatening thromboembolism or thrombosis. The risk of thromboembolic events should be evaluated for each patient and prophylaxis initiated where appropriate.
  - Young women with hypertension, hyperlipidemia, obesity, diabetes, or prolonged immobility may be predisposed to experiencing adverse effects.

Follow-Up

- For persistent vaginal bleeding despite intervention as outlined above consider other causes: coagulopathy; vaginitis, cervicitis, trauma, tumor, pregnancy; nongenital bleeding (rectal, urethral); precocious puberty.
- The time to return of normal menses is variable following discontinuation of menses suppression.

Tips

- Beware of thromboembolic risks of oral contraceptives in patients who become bedridden postop or following intensive chemotherapy.

References

Chiarelli AM, Marrett LD, Darlington G. Early menopause and infertility in females after treatment for childhood cancer diagnosed in 1964–1988 in Ontario, Canada. *Am J Epidemiol*. 1999;150:245–254.

Seli E, Tangir J. Fertility preservation options for female patients with malignancies. *Curr Opin Obstet Gynecol*. 2005;17:299–308.

Whitehead E, Shalets S, Blackedge G, et al. The effect of combination chemotherapy on ovarian function in women treated for Hodgkin's disease. *Cancer*. 1983;52:988–993.

c h a p t e r   1 0

Mucositis

Angela Punnett

Outline

- Introduction
- Etiology
- Prevention
- Clinical Presentation
- Initial Management
- Follow-up

Introduction

- Painful condition that interferes with patient function and tolerance of therapy.
- Occurs in 40 % of all patients receiving chemotherapy.

Etiology

- Chemotherapy, radiation, and myelosuppression.
- Risk factors: hematologic malignancy, pediatric population, poor oral health, specific chemotherapy agents (alkylating agents, antimetabolites, antibiotics), combination therapy, dose and schedule of chemotherapy/radiation, hematopoietic stem cell transplant recipients.

Prevention

- Maintain good oral hygiene to reduce risk and severity of mucositis.
- Perform regular dental assessments and proactive dental treatment in consultation with oncology.
- Remove orthodontic bands prior to chemotherapy.
- Encourage use of regular soft toothbrush (according to age/size), and teeth brushing 2–3 times/day.
- Dental floss may be used if patients, or their caregivers, have experience preceding diagnosis and demonstrate proper technique.
- If mucositis develops and/or the patient is unable to use a soft toothbrush due to bleeding, use baking soda rinses (2–3 times/day); for children who are unable to spit out the mouthwash, give swish/swallow water rinses instead; for very young children, gently clean teeth and gums with a clean damp washcloth wrapped around a finger.
- Sponge foam sticks are not as effective in removing bacterial plaque.
- Avoid alcohol-based mouthwashes, full-strength peroxide solutions, and any irritant to the oral mucosa (spicy or acidic food, alcohol).

- Chlorhexidine 0.12 % rinse has been used for prevention but can be irritating and efficacy is controversial.
- Baking soda rinse is recommended after vomiting, ideally before brushing.

Clinical Presentation

- Erythema, inflammation, ulceration, and hemorrhage in the mouth and throat.
- A number of grading systems exist for assessment of mucositis in adults, but there is limited evaluation of instruments in children.
- Issues specific to the pediatric assessment: illumination, appropriate visualization of the oral cavity, and uncooperative child.
- Two commonly used grading systems:
  - Functional/Symptomatic Grading System (CTCAE version 3.0).
    - Grade 1: Minimal symptoms, normal diet; respiratory symptoms but not interfering with function.
    - Grade 2: Symptomatic but can eat and swallow modified diet; respiratory symptoms interfering with function but not interfering with ADLs.
    - Grade 3: Symptomatic and unable to adequately aliment or hydrate orally; respiratory symptoms interfering with ADL.
    - Grade 4: Symptoms associated with life-threatening consequences.
    - Grade 5: Death.
  - Clinical appearance of oral mucosa (WHO):
    - Grade 1: Soreness +/− erythema.
    - Grade 2: Erythema, ulcers; patient can swallow solid food.

- Grade 3: Erythema, ulcers; patient cannot swallow solid food.
- Grade 4: Mucositis to the extent that alimentation is not possible.

- Differential diagnosis: bacterial, viral, and fungal infection.
- Typical oral flora are often a source of infection, but opportunistic organisms may cause local infection and lead to sepsis.

Initial Management

- No specific practical guidelines for children.
- Rule out and treat any infection:
  - Degree and duration of neutropenia determines the incidence and severity of infection.
  - Oral infection may present only with evidence of inflammation.
  - Treatment of oral thrush (*C. albicans*):
    - Fluconazole.
  - With significant ulceration or potential infectious contact:
    - Swab for herpes viruses PCR (use NP swab).
    - Treat with IV or PO acyclovir as appropriate.
- Continue good oral hygiene as above.
- Consider topical pain management:
  - SickKids mouthwash for pain (lidocaine viscous 12 mg/ml in sugar-free Kool-Aid) 5 ml swish/spit QID PRN, or viscous lidocaine applied to affected area(s) QID PRN. Note: Swallowing can impair gag reflex and increase risk of aspiration.
  - Benzydamine (Tantum) rinse swish/spit QID PRN. Contains alcohol and may cause severe stinging.

- Consider systemic pain management:
  - Oral: Codeine, morphine (avoid acetaminophen since it will mask a fever).
  - Inpatient/IV: Morphine boluses or infusion.
- Severe cases of mucositis require admission for analgesia and nutritional support.

Follow-Up

- Severe mucositis may necessitate a change to patient cancer treatment plan. Document mucositis severity, and review treatment protocol guidelines for any modification of chemotherapy.
- Consider prophylactic acyclovir for recurrent HSV-related mucositis during periods of neutropenia, and as per patient's treatment plan.

References

American Academy of Pediatric Dentistry. *Clinical Guideline on Dental Management of Pediatric Patients Receiving Chemotherapy, Hematopoietic Cell Transplantation, and/or Radiation*. Chicago, IL: American Academy of Pediatric Dentistry; 2004.

Keefe DM, Schubert MM, Elting LS, et al. Updated clinical practice guidelines for the prevention and treatment of mucositis. *Cancer*. 2007;109: 820–831.

Silverman S. Diagnosis and management of oral mucositis. *Support Oncol*. 2006;5(2):S1:13–21.

Tomlinson D, Judd P, Hendershot E, et al. Measurement of oral mucositis in children: a review of the literature. *Support Care Cancer*. 2007;15(11): 1251–1258.

c h a p t e r   1 1

Neurological Complications

Vicky R. Breakey, Ute Bartels, and Rand Askalan

Outline

- Introduction
- Clinical Presentations
- Specific Syndromes

Introduction

- Neurological complications occur in 5–10% of children with malignancy.
- Most common causes: Infections, drug toxicity, neoplasm, vascular, and metabolic.
- Common clinical presentations: Seizures, headache, altered level of consciousness, and focal neurological deficit.
- Mortality: Up to 30%. Long-term morbidities include epilepsy and cognitive impairment.

Clinical Presentations

Seizures

- Most common central nervous system (CNS) complication in pediatric cancer; mostly partial simple seizures with or without secondary generalization, rarely partial complex or absence seizures.

Etiology

- Infectious:
  - Meningitis, encephalitis, brain abscesses.
  - Common pathogens: Aspergillus, Streptococci, Enterovirus, and Herpes Zoster.
- Drug toxicity: Intrathecal and/or systemic chemotherapeutic drugs, especially methotrexate, vincristine, ifosfamide, cisplatin.
- Neoplasm:
  - Primary CNS neoplasm: New diagnosis, relapse, progression or intratumoral bleeding.
  - CNS leukemia.
  - Brain metastases.
- Vascular:
  - Arterial ischemic stroke due to hypercoagulability or inherited thrombophilia.
  - Sinus venous thrombosis associated with asparaginase therapy.
  - Intracranial hemorrhage: Increased with thrombocytopenia, coagulopathy/DIC, hyperleukocytosis.
- Metabolic disturbances: Hyponatremia, hypocalcemia, hypomagnesemia, and hypoglycemia.
- Posterior reversible encephalopathy syndrome (PRES): See "Specific Syndromes" section.

Initial Management

- Assess/manage airway and facilitate breathing; apply 100% oxygen by mask.
- Maintain a safe environment to prevent injury; if possible bring patient to lateral position.
- Ensure adequate intravenous access.
- Urgently check electrolytes, calcium, magnesium, glucose, CBC, INR/PTT, venous blood gases, and request blood cultures if patient is febrile.
- If seizure lasts > 5 minutes, treat pharmacologically with a stepwise approach:
  1. Lorazepam 0.1 mg/kg IV (max 4 mg), repeat once after 5 minutes if no response.
  2. Phenobarbitol 20 mg/kg IV (max 800 mg) as slow infusion over 20 minutes; monitor for respiratory depression/apnea.
  3. Phenytoin 20 mg/kg IV (max 1 g) as slow infusion over 20 minutes; monitor for bradycardia and hypotension.
  4. Paraldehyde 100% 0.2–0.3 ml/kg (200–400 mg/kg, max 5 ml) per rectum over 15 minutes; may repeat once.
  5. For neurotoxicity secondary to ifosfamide, consider use of methylene blue.
- For persistent seizure, hemodynamic instability, or difficulty maintaining airway, consult pediatric critical care team.
- Urgent CT head scan if history and/or physical exam suggests focal lesion or if there is evidence of increased intracranial pressure (ICP) (in practice, at the Hospital for Sick Children-Toronto, we obtain a CT on all our patients who present with a seizure).

Further Work-Up

- After the seizure has stopped, consider neuroimaging (CT, MRI), EEG, and lumbar puncture (LP) to determine etiology.
- If patient has received asparaginase obtain a CT-venogram and/or an MR-angiography (MRA)/MR-venography (MRV).
- For suspected infection, obtain blood, urine, and CSF cultures; nasal and throat swabs; PCR for viral studies: Enterovirus, Varicella-Zoster (VZV), and Herpes simplex virus (HSV); and tissue biopsy as indicated.

Follow-Up

- If further seizures develop, consider referral to a pediatric neurologist and initiation of therapy with anticonvulsants.
- Proceed with caution when prescribing anticonvulsants as they may interact with chemotherapy, suppress bone marrow function, or cause liver toxicity.
- Preferred anticonvulsants in this patient population include gabapentin, levetiracetam, and clobazam.
- Consider sublingual/rectal benzodiazepines at home for seizures lasting greater than five minutes.
- Parent/patient education: Precautions for epileptics around bathing, swimming, and driving.

Headache

- Common complaint in pediatric oncology patients.
- Important to identify serious headaches with underlying pathology; usually they are associated with signs of increased ICP and are persistent and difficult to treat.

Etiology

- Infectious: Meningitis, encephalitis, brain abscesses, and fungal infections.
- Drugs:
  - Intrathecal chemotherapy.
  - Systemic chemotherapy: vincristine, cytarabine, etoposide, asparaginase, doxorubicin, cyclophosphamide, and rituximab.
  - Drugs causing increased ICP: Retinoic acid (ATRA syndrome, see Chapter 2), cyclosporine A, amphotericin-B, ciprofloxacin, tetracycline.
  - Other medications: Narcotics, antiemetics (ondansetron, granisetron).
- Neoplasm:
  - Primary CNS malignancy.
  - Brain metastasis (uncommon in children).
  - CNS leukemia, cerebral chloroma (AML).
- Vascular: Stroke, intracranial hemorrhage, and sinus venous thrombosis.
- Idiopathic intracranial hypertension (pseudotumor cerebri).
- Iatrogenic:
  - Postlumbar puncture headache.
  - Postcranial irradiation.
- Psychogenic: Depression, anxiety.

Management

- First, rule out increased ICP and other serious causes.
- Supportive care:
  - Analgesia may include oral codeine or morphine; avoid administering acetaminophen for headaches in neutropenic patients as it may mask a fever, and avoid NSAIDS due to the potential of platelet dysfunction.

○ Caffeine tablets can be helpful for post-LP headaches.

○ Consider consulting psychiatry or psychology if indicated, especially in teenagers.

Increased ICP

- Symptoms:
  ○ Headache (often worse at waking), nausea/vomiting.
  ○ Visual disturbances.
  ○ Lethargy, irritability, and decreasing level of consciousness as pressure increases.
- Signs:
  ○ Papilledema, bulging fontanel.
  ○ Cranial nerve VI palsy (often referred to as a "false localizing sign").
  ○ Cushing's triad: Increased systolic blood pressure with wide pulse pressure, bradycardia, and abnormal respiratory pattern.
  ○ Unequal/unresponsive pupils, sun-setting eyes at advanced stage (imminent risk of herniation).
- Urgent management:
  ○ Fundoscopy and neuroimaging essential.
  ○ Neurosurgical consult for surgical intervention (extraventricular drain, ventriculostomy, decompression if space-occupying lesion).
  ○ Notify intensive care unit.
  ○ Elevate head of bed to 30°, keep head midline, and avoid hyperthermia.
  ○ Dexamethasone 0.1–0.25 mg/kg IV q 6 h.
  ○ In cases of GCS < 8, intubation is required:
    ■ Laryngoscopy and intubation may result in further elevations in intracranial pressure that can be attenuated using lidocaine, opioids, or benzodiazepines and by avoiding depolarizing neuromuscu-

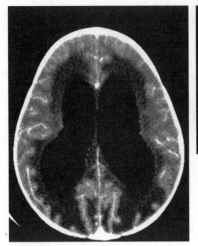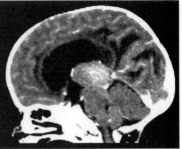

Figure 11-1 Hydrocephalus and increased intracranial pressure in a 1 year old boy with increasing head circumference, ataxia, and nystagmus. Courtesy of Diagnostic Imaging, The Hospital for Sick Children, Toronto, Canada.

lar blockers. This should be done in consultation with a pediatric anesthetist/intensivist.

- ■ Mildly hyperventilate to $Paco_2$ 30–35 mmHg.
- ○ Maintain cerebral perfusion pressure (CPP = mean arterial pressure − intracranial pressure); consider ICP monitoring if unstable.
- ○ If neurological assessment and brain imaging are normal, consider LP to check CSF opening pressure (diagnostic for increased ICP if > 25 cm H_2O).
- ○ For pseudotumor cerebri, repetitive LPs or treatment with acetazolamide may relieve symptoms (see Chapter 2).
- • Follow-up:
  - ○ Regular ophthalmologic assessment: Monitor for recurrent or chronic increased ICP to prevent optic atrophy and visual loss.

Altered Level of Consciousness

- Impairment of perception and behavior, decreased awareness of self and environment, spectrum from somnolence to coma.

Etiology

- Infectious: Encephalitis, septicemia, other severe infections.
- Drugs: Narcotics, overdose/ingestion/intoxication.
- Neoplasm: Cerebral tumors.
- Vascular: Stroke, intracranial hemorrhage, and sinus venous thrombosis.
- Metabolic: Hypoglycemia, uremia, hypernatremia, liver failure.
- Psychiatric: Acute psychosis, ICU psychosis.
- Others: Increased ICP, shunt malfunction, posterior reversible encephalopathy syndrome (PRES).

Initial Management

- Resuscitation as indicated.
- Clinical assessment: Modified Glasgow Coma Scale (GCS; Table 11-1).
- Neurological examination; look for evidence of trauma, increased ICP, localizing signs.
- If focal findings on physical exam, consider subdural hematoma, intracerebral hemorrhage, tumor, abscess, infarction, herpes encephalitis, or focal seizure.
- Diagnostic work-up:
  - Blood: CBC, electrolytes, blood gases, creatinine, BUN, liver enzymes, ammonium, INR/PTT, toxin screen (including acetaminophen, ASA, alcohol levels).
  - Urine: Culture, toxin screen.

Table 11-1 Modified Glasgow Coma Scale.

	Score	< 1 Year Old	> 1 Year Old
Eye Opening	4	Spontaneously	Spontaneously
	3	To shout	To verbal command
	2	To pain	To pain
	1	No response	No response
Motor response	6	Obeys	Obeys
	5	Localizes pain	Localizes pain
	4	Flexion withdrawal	Flexion withdrawal
	3	Decorticate	Decorticate
	2	Decerebrate	Decerebrate
	1	No response	No response

	Score	0–23 Months	2–5 Years	> 5 Years
Verbal response	5	Smiles, coos, cries	Appropriate words, phrases	Oriented and converses
	4	Cries	Inappropriate words	Disoriented and converses
	3	Inappropriate cry, screams	Cries or screams	Inappropriate words
	2	Grunts	Grunts	Incomprehensible sounds
	1	No response	No response	No response

Source: Courtesy of Critical Care Unit, The Hospital for Sick Children, Toronto, Canada

○ CSF: Protein, glucose, cytology, gram stain, culture, assessment of opening pressure. (LP is contraindicated if patient is comatose, hemodynamically unstable, has localizing signs, evidence of increased ICP, or coagulopathy.)

○ CT head; urgent if focal neurological deficit.

○ Consult pediatric neurology and consider EEG.

○ Definitive management and follow-up vary with underlying etiology.

Focal Neurological Deficit

Etiology

- Infectious: Brain abscess, disseminated CNS infection with seeding to spinal cord.
- Drugs:
  ○ Chemotherapy-associated peripheral neuropathy (vincristine, vinblastine, cisplatin, arsenic).
  ○ Chemotherapy-associated myelopathy: Intrathecal methotrexate and cytarabine.
- Neoplasm: CNS tumors, metastases, leukemic chloroma.
- Vascular:
  ○ Stroke, intracranial hemorrhage.
  ○ Epidural or subdural hemorrhage following LP (in patients with coagulopathy).
- Other: Cranial nerve palsies, most commonly CN VI, may result in secondary to increased ICP.

Specific Syndromes

Acute Spinal Cord Compression

- *Absolute emergency*!
- Incidence: 5 % of children with cancer at presentation.

Etiology

- Solid tumors: Ewing's sarcoma most common, followed by neuroblastoma, osteosarcoma, and rhabdomyosarcoma (rarely lymphoma or leukemia).
- Brain tumor metastases or primary spinal tumors.

Clinical Presentation

- Often presents with localized pain followed by progressive weakness, sensory deficits, paresis, and incontinence.

Initial Management

- Early consultation with a pediatric oncologist and neurosurgeon is essential.

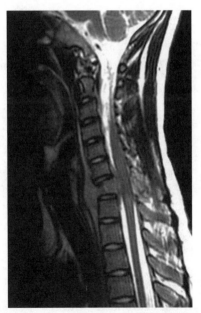

Figure 11-2 Spinal MRI shows mass at C7/T1 level in a 15 year old boy who presented with acute onset of bilateral leg weakness and parasthesias.
Courtesy of Diagnostic Imaging, The Hospital for Sick Children, Toronto, Canada.

- Immediate MRI (gadolinium enhanced) indicated if patient is nonambulatory; otherwise, it should be completed within 24 hours of presentation.
- Dexamethasone may be utilized to decrease swelling:
  - 1–2 mg/kg/day IV divided q 6 h for rapidly progressive deficits.
  - 0.25–0.5 mg/kg PO q 6 h for subacute presentation.
  - If lymphoma is within the differential diagnosis, a biopsy must be obtained within first 24 hours of steroid therapy.
- Surgery consultation for decompression and/or to obtain tissue if diagnosis is uncertain.
- Urgent radiotherapy can be beneficial if tumor is suspected to be radiosensitive.

Follow-Up

- Further therapy for malignancy, which may include chemotherapy, radiation, and surgery.
- Requires long-term follow-up with a pediatric oncologist, neurosurgeon, and orthopedist.
- Neurological function at presentation is best predictor of long-term functional outcome.

Vincristine-Induced Peripheral Neuropathy

- Vast majority of peripheral neuropathy in children with cancer is secondary to vincristine, and it develops to some degree in almost all patients.

Clinical Presentation

- Severe jaw pain can occur within a few hours of the first dose of vincristine.
- Peripheral parasthesias and loss of deep tendon reflexes are common and may occur at any time during therapy.

- With prolonged therapy and/or high doses, wrist and foot drop may occur, followed by a slapping gait, difficulty in walking and/or unbuttoning shirts.
- Cranial nerve deficits include vocal cord paresis or paralysis, ocular motor nerve dysfunction, and facial nerve palsies.
- Autonomic neuropathy: Constipation, abdominal pain, and ileus.
- Central neuropathy: Headache, dizziness, seizures, SIADH, psychosis.

Initial Management

- Jaw pain can be treated with codeine or morphine; avoid acetaminophen in neutropenic patients as it may mask a fever.
- Peripheral neuropathy often necessitates reduction in dose of vincristine and may lead to cessation of usage.
- Glutamine: Promising treatment for vincristine-induced neuropathy; a phase II study is currently underway at the NCI.

Follow-Up

- Most peripheral neuropathy is reversible, but may persist for months.
- Rarely symptoms may be disabling, necessitating referral to a pediatric neurologist, pain specialist, physiotherapy, or orthotics (for foot drop or limping).

Posterior Reversible Encephalopathy Syndrome (PRES)

- A clinico-radiological phenomenon associated with a variety of medical conditions: cancer, hematological diseases, connective tissue disorders, renal diseases, and eclampsia.

- Pathophysiology: Unclear but triggers include hypertension and immunosuppressive/cytotoxic drugs: tacrolimus, cytarabine, methotrexate, vincristine.
- Despite being rare, PRES is becoming increasingly recognized and diagnosed in pediatric cancer patients.
- Contrary to the name, the sequelae are not always reversible and may include residual changes on imaging, persistent abnormal EEG, and epilepsy.

Clinical Presentation

- Acute headache, seizures, altered mental status, hypertension, and/or visual problems.
- Neuroimaging: Bilateral white matter lesions, usually in the parietal and occipital lobes.

Initial Management

- Seizure management as above.
- Treat/prevent exacerbating factors of PRES, e.g., concomitant hypomagnesemia.
- Exclude elevated ICP as cause of hypertension, then treat high blood pressure (BP):
  - Nifedipine 0.15 mg/kg PO q 4 h (max 10 mg/dose, given as bite and swallow) *or*
  - Hydralazine 0.15–0.8 mg/kg/dose IV q 4 h (max 25 mg/dose).
  - If BP remains uncontrolled, consider infusion (ICU consultation should be considered):
    - Labetolol 0.4–3 mg/kg/h continuous infusion (contraindicated in asthmatics and patients in congestive heart failure) *or*
    - Nitroprusside 0.25–8 micrograms/kg/min continuous infusion (avoid in renal failure and elevated ICP).

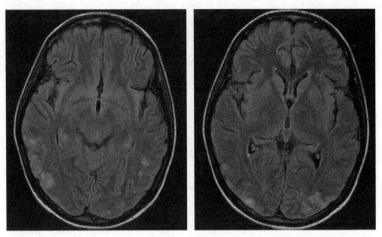

Figure 11-3 A 14-year-old girl with Non-Hodgkin's Lymphoma undergoing induction chemotherapy presented with acute headache, hypertension, and seizure. MRI was consistent with PRES.
Courtesy of Diagnostic Imaging, The Hospital for Sick Children, Toronto, Canada.

Follow-Up

- Consider changing or holding chemotherapeutic agent (most likely to be the cause).
- If there are no further seizures and EEG/neuroimaging revert to normal, consider withdrawal of anticonvulsants.

References

Brannon Morris E, Laningham FH, Sandlund JT et al. Posterior reversible encephalopathy syndrome in children with cancer. *Pediatr Blood Cancer*. 2007;48:152–159.

Huang LT, Hsaio CC, Weng HH, et al. Neurological complications of pediatric systemic malignancies. *J Formos Med Assoc*. 1996;95:209–212.

Schmidt K, Schultz AS, Debatin K-M, et al. CNS complications in children receiving chemotherapy or hematopoetic stem cell transplantation: retrospective analysis and clinical study of survivors. *Pediatr Blood Cancer*. 2008;50:331–336.

c h a p t e r   1 2

Nutritional Support

Gloria J. Green and Angela Punnett

Outline

- Malnutrition
- Nutritional Assessment
- Initial Management
- Follow-Up

Malnutrition

Etiology

- Malnutrition may be present at the diagnosis of cancer and/or develop as a result of treatment.
- The prevalence of malnutrition ranges from 6% to 50% and is associated with tumor type and extent of metastatic disease.
- Nutritional high-risk tumors: Stage IV neuroblastoma/ Wilm's/Ewings, relapsed solid tumors or leukemias, high-risk medulloblastoma, acute Myeloid leukemia (AML).

- The cause of malnutrition is multifactorial and may include decreased nutrient intake and/or absorption, increased losses, and a catabolic state with increased energy requirements.

Complications

- Poor nutrition increases susceptibility to infection, decreases tolerance of chemotherapy, and is associated with decreased survival and prolonged hospitalizations.
- Adequate nutrition is required during periods of rapid growth, and suboptimal nutrition can lead to growth retardation.
- Corticosteroids (frequently used as part of chemotherapy treatment or as antiemetic agents) are associated with hyperglycemia, fluid retention, hyperphagia, weight gain, and in the longer term low bone mineral density.

Nutritional Assessment

- All patients require ongoing nutritional assessment and monitoring:
  - Anthropometric measurements of weight, height, calculation of percent weight for height (%WFH), and percent weight change.
  - In children with solid tumors, the tumor mass itself may cause body weight to be an inaccurate predictor of nutritional status.
  - Triceps skin fold measurements (TSF) and midarm circumference (MAC) to assess fat store status and somatic muscle mass have been shown to be useful in children with cancer.
  - Dietary history and review of calorie counts.

Initial Management

- Efforts should be made to meet nutritional needs orally. See Figure 12-1. Other nutritional interventions include enteral and parenteral nutrition.

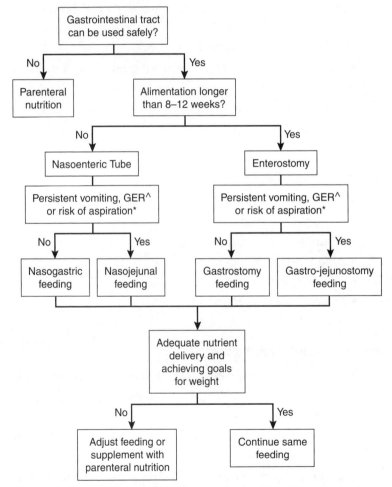

Figure 12-1 Algorithm for Selecting the Route of Nutritional Support.
^ Gastroesophageal reflux.
* Despite treatment with prokinetic and acid inhibitory agents.
Taken with permission from "Guidelines for the Administration of Enteral and Parenteral Nutrition in Paediatrics." *SickKids*, 3rd ed. June 2007.

Enteral Nutrition

Indications

- Enteral tube feeding should be initiated when a child is unable to meet nutrient or fluid needs orally.
- Potential situations include anorexia associated with the disease or treatment, dysphagia, unsafe to feed orally secondary to tumor location, and radiation treatment affecting the integrity of the mouth/gut.
- Enteral feeding is preferred to parenteral feeding whenever possible. It maintains gut mucosal integrity, prevents pancreatic and biliary flow dysfunction, has fewer complications, and is lower in cost.

Contraindications for Use

- Hemodynamic instability.
- Persistent vomiting or diarrhea.
- Acute abdominal distention.
- Upper gastrointestinal bleeding.
- Bowel obstruction or ileus.
- Typhlitis/pneumatosis intestinalis.

Enteral Tube Feeding Route

- Nasogastric (NG) tubes: Check platelets (recommend platelets $> 50 \times 10^9/l$), absolute neutrophil count (recommend $> 0.5 \times 10^9/l$) before insertion.
- Nasojejunal (NJ) tubes are more difficult to position and require radiological placement.
- Long-term use of NG or NJ tubes is associated with esophagitis and/or gastroesophageal reflux (GER).
- If tube feeding is required for greater than 8–12 weeks, gastrostomy (G) tube placement should be considered.

- A gastrojejunostomy (GJ) tube may be warranted if a G tube has been unsuccessful in preventing GER and/or aspiration pneumonia. These tubes are usually placed by an interventional radiologist.
- GJ tubes require continuous feeding administration (cannot do intermittent or bolus feeds).
- Guidelines for initiating and advancing tube feedings in infants and children (see Figure 12-2).

Age	Initial hourly infusion	Daily increases	Goal
Continuous and continuous nocturnal infusion			
Preterm	1–2mL/kg/h	1 mL q feed	120–200 mL/kg/d
0–1 year	10–20 mL/h or 1–2 mL/kg/h	5–10 mL/8h or 1 mL/kg/h	21–54 mL/h or 6 mL/kg/h
1–6 years	20–30 mL/h or 2–3 mL/kg/h	10–15 mL/8 h or 1 mL/kg/h	71–92 mL/h or 4–5 mL/kg/h
6–14 years	30–40 mL/h or 1 mL/kg/h	15–20 mL/8 h or 0.5 mL/kg/h	108–130 mL/h or 3–4 mL/kg/h
>14 years	50 mL/h or 0.5–1 mL/kg/h	25 mL/8 h or 0.4–0.5 mL/kg/h	125 mL/h
Intermittent infusion			
Preterm >1200g	2–4 mL/kg/feed		
0–1year	60–80 mL q 4 h or 10–15 mL/kg/feed	20–40 mL q 4 h	80–240 mL q 4 h or 20–30 mL/kg/feed
1–6 years	80–120 mL q 4 h or 5–10 mL/kg/feed	40–60 mL q 4 h	280–375 mL q 4 h or 15–20 mL/kg/feed
6–14 years	120–160 mL q 4 h or 3–5 mL/kg/feed	60–80 mL q 4 h	430–520 mL q 4 h or 10–20 mL/kg/feed
>14 years	200 mL q 4 h or 3 mL/kg/feed	100 mL q 4 h	500 mL q 4 h or 10 mL/kg/feed

Figure 12-2   Guidelines for Initiating and Advancing Tube Feedings in Infants and Children.

NOTE: Rates expressed per kg body weight are useful for small-for-age patients

Taken with permission from "Guidelines for the Administration of enteral and Pareneral Nutrition in Paediatrics." *SickKids*, 3rd ed. June 2007 (Source adapted from Wilson S.E. Pediatric Enteral Feeding. In: Pediatric Nutrition, Theory and Practice. Grand RJ, Sutphen JL, et al, eds. Toronto, Ont: Butterworth; 1987).

Parenteral Nutrition (PN)

- May be used as a primary source of nutrition, providing full nutrition support, or may supplement enteral nutrition.

Indications

- Nonfunctioning GI tract (mucositis, typhlitis, diarrhea, nausea/vomiting, ileus, etc.).
- Inadequate intake for 2–3 days infants/young child, 4–5 days older child/adolescent.
- Recent weight loss > 5% usual body weight (UBW) and insufficient enteral intake.

Contraindications

- Medically unstable.
- Requirement for < 3 days.
- Sole purpose of electrolyte replacement.

Ordering PN

Guidelines provided below are for the initiation of PN. Wherever possible, consultation with the unit dietician is recommended at initiation and required for ongoing management of PN.

- Energy requirements are estimated to be approximately 10–15% less than enteral feeding because gastrointestinal energy losses and the cost of digestion are minimal. Therefore basal metabolic rate (BMR) is used instead of the DRI (see Table 12-1).
- Protein is ideally not used for energy but for maintaining or promoting lean body mass. To ensure that amino acids are being used for anabolism, a minimum amount must be supplied with the right proportion of nonprotein calories (see Table 12-2).

Estimated energy requirement (EER)* (kcal/kg/d)					
		Physical activity level (PAL)+			
Age	**Sex**	**Sedentary**	**Low active**	**Active**	**Very active**
Infants (mo)					
0–2	M	107			
	F	104–102			
3–6	M	95–82			
	F	95–82			
7–9	M	79–80			
	F	80			
10–20	M	79–82			
	F	82			
21–35	M	82–83			
	F	83			
Children (y)					
3–4	M	81–75	93–86	104–97	117–109
	F	78–72	89–83	100–94	118–111
5–6	M	69–64	80–74	90–84	103–97
	F	66–62	77–72	87–82	104–97
7–8	M	60–57	70–66	80–75	92–87
	F	57–53	67–62	75–71	90–85
9–10	M	54–50	63–59	71–67	83–78
	F	49–45	57–53	65–60	78–72
11–12	M	47–44	55–52	64–60	74–70
	F	41–39	49–46	56–63	67–64
13–14	M	42–41	50–48	57–56	67–64
	F	37–35	44–41	50–47	60–57
15–16	M	40–38	47–45	54–52	62–60
	F	33–32	40–38	45–44	55–54
17–18	M	37–36	43–42	50–49	58–57
	F	31–30	37–36	43–42	52–51

Figure 12-3   Summary of Estimated Energy Requirement (EER) for Infants and Children.

+ PAL for infants not determined

* EER (kcal/kg) calculated based on equations on p.19 dividend by reference weights.

Taken with permission from "Guidelines for the Administration of Enteral and Parenteral Nutrition in Paediatrics." *SickKids*, 3rd ed. June 2007.

Table 12-1 Calculating parenteral energy requirements: Equations for predicting basal metabolic rate from body weight (W).

Age Range (yr)	Kcal/day	
	Males	**Females**
0–3	60.9W − 54	61.0W − 51
3–10	22.7W + 495	22.5W − 499
10–18	17.5W + 651	12.2W + 746

NOTE: Does not account for physical activity, growth, or any specific nutritional stressors (i.e., fever, sepsis).

Situation	Activity Factor
Paralyzed, comatose	0.8–1.0
Confined to bed	1.2
Sedentary	1.5
Normal activity	1.7

Source: With permission from "Guidelines for the Administration of Enteral and Parenteral Nutrition in Paediatrics." *SickKids*, 3rd ed. 2007 (adapted from World Health Organization. *Energy and Protein Requirements*. Technical Report Series 724, Geneva, Switzerland; 1985).

Table 12-2 Guidelines for administration of parenteral amino acids.

	0–1 yr	1–12 yr	> 12 yr
Initial Dose (g/kg/d)	1.0–1.5	1.5–2.0	1.5
Advance Daily (g/kg/d)	1.0	—	—
Recommended (g/kg/d)	2.5–3.0	1.5–2.0	1.5–2.0

Source: Taken with permission from "Guidelines for the Administration of Enteral and Parenteral Nutrition in Paediatrics." *SickKids*, 3rd ed. 2007.

- Carbohydrate: Dextrose supplies the majority of non-protein calories and osmolality in parenteral nutrition solutions. Unlike enteral glucose, this form provides 3.4 kcals/g of carbohydrate. *Solutions greater than 12.5% dextrose should not be infused in a peripheral line.* Carbohydrate should be initiated in a stepwise fashion (see Table 12-3).

- Fat: Parenteral lipids (20%, 30%) are isotonic, provide a concentrated source of calories, and can prevent or reverse essential fatty acid deficiency. Lipids should be infused over 24 hours for better tolerance and advanced in a stepwise fashion (see Table 12-4). Tolerance is measured by an intralipid level (goal < 1.0 g/l) or triglycerides/cholesterol levels. Intravenous lipids are contraindicated for patients with an allergy to egg.

- Fluid and electrolyte management should be individualized (see Tables 12-5 and 12-6). Fluid losses (e.g., intractable diarrhea, vomiting, ostomy output) should be replaced through a separate replacement IV source.

Table 12-3   Guidelines for administration of parenteral dextrose.

	Full Term/ Children	Adolescent
Initial Dose (mg/kg/d)	7–9	3–5
Advance Daily* (mg/kg/d)	1–3	1–3
Recommended + (mg/kg/d)	11–12	5–8

* Rate of advancement is determined by glucose tolerance.
+ Maximum intake will be determined by both tolerance and route of administration.
Source: Taken with permission from "Guidelines for the Administration of Enteral and Parenteral Nutrition in Paediatrics." *SickKids*, 3rd ed. 2007.

Table 12-4 Guidelines for administration of parenteral lipids.

	Full Term	Older Children/ Adolescent
Initial Dose (g/kg/d)	1.0	1.0
Advance Daily (g/kg/d)	0.5–1.0	0.5–1.0
Recommended (g/kg/d)	4.0	2.0–4.0

Source: Taken with permission from "Guidelines for the Administration of Enteral and Parenteral Nutrition in Paediatrics." *SickKids*, 3rd ed. 2007.

Table 12-5 Maintenance fluid requirements calculations.

Patient Weight	Daily Maintenance Fluid Requirements
< 10 kg	100 ml/kg
10–20 kg	1000 ml + 50 ml for each kg > 10 kg
> 20 kg	1500 ml + 20 ml for each kg > 20 kg

Source: Taken with permission from "Guidelines for the Administration of Enteral and Parenteral Nutrition in Paediatrics." *SickKids*, 3rd ed. 2007.

- Certain incompatible medications make it necessary to cycle the total PN volume over a shorter period. Careful consideration should be given to the total fluid and nutrients given.
- Labs to be monitored and frequency of monitoring:
  ○ For stable patients:
    ■ Glucose at start of therapy, and × 2/wk.
    ■ Electrolytes at start of therapy, and × 2/wk.
    ■ Intralipid level or triglycerides/cholesterol × 2/wk.

Table 12-6 Daily electrolyte and mineral requirements for pediatric patients.

	Preterm Neonates	Infants/Children	Adolescents & Children > 50 kg
Sodium	2–5 mmol/kg	2–5 mmol/kg	1–2 mmol/kg
Potassium	2–4 mmol/kg	2–4 mmol/kg	1–2 mmol/kg
Chloride	As needed to maintain acid–base balance	As needed to maintain acid–base balance	As needed to maintain acid–base balance
Calcium	1–2 mmol/kg	0.25–2 mmol/kg	5–10 mmol/d
Phosphorus	1–2 mmol/kg	0.5–2 mmol/kg	10–40 mmol/d
Magnesium	0.15–0.25 mmol/kg	0.15–0.25 mmol/kg	5–15 mmol/d
Acetate	As needed to maintain acid–base balance	As needed to maintain acid–base balance	As needed to maintain acid–base balance

Source: Taken with permission from "Guidelines for the Administration of Enteral and Parenteral Nutrition in Paediatrics." *SickKids*, 3rd ed. 2007 (Source adapted from the *ASPEN Nutrition Support Manual*, 2nd. ed. American Society for Parenteral and Enteral Nutrition; 2005).

- Urea, phosphate, calcium, conj/unconj bilirubin, albumin, Mg at start of therapy and × 2/wk.
- AST, ALT, Alk Phos, Creat, acid base, at start of therapy and × 2/wk.
  ○ For unstable patients, such as with liver or renal dysfunction caused by disease or side effects of medications/chemotherapeutic agents:
    - Increased potassium needs (amphotericin), increased Mg needs (cisplatin), hyperglycemia secondary to steroids → more frequent monitoring may be warranted.
- If adjustments are made to PN solution as a result of abnormal lab results → more frequent monitoring is indicated for tailoring of solution and rates until normalized.

Follow-Up

- Long-term follow-up of growth and nutritional status is important to monitor for late effects of cancer therapy.
- Obesity has been identified as a significant morbidity of some cancer therapies; counseling around appropriate nutrition and activity levels is necessary.

References

Acra S, Rollins C. Principles and guidelines for parenteral nutrition in children. *Pediatr Annals*. 1999;28:113–20.

ASPEN Board of Directors. Guidelines for the use of parenteral and enteral nutrition in adult and pediatric patients. *JPEN*. 2002;26(1 Suppl):9–16A.

Baugh N, Recuper MA, Kerner JA. Nutritional requirements for pediatric patients. In: Christensen ML, ed. *A.S.P.E.N. Nutrition Support Practice Manual*. Silver Spring, MD: American Society of Parenteral and Enteral Nutrition;1998:1–13.

Pearce CB, Duncan HD. Enteral feeding. Nasogastric, nasojejunal, percutaneous endoscopic gastrostomy, or jejunostomy: its indications and limitations. *Postgrad Med J.* 2002;78:198–204.

SickKids Nutrition Team Members. Guidelines for the administration of enteral and parenteral nutrition in paediatrics. *SickKids.* 3rd ed. Toronto, Ontario, Canada: The Hospital for Sick Kids; 2007.

Wilson SE, Dietz WH, Grand RJ. An algorithm for pediatric enteral alimentation. *Pediatr Ann.* 1987;16(3):233–240.

chapter 13

Pain Control in Pediatric Oncology

Jocelyne Volpe and Basem Naser

Outline

- Introduction
- Incidence
- Etiology
- Assessment
- Barriers to Good Pain Control
- Management

Introduction

- Pain is an unpleasant sensory experience and an emotional experience associated with actual or potential tissue damage. Pain is the subjective experience of the patient.

- Pain is the most debilitating symptom for children with cancer.
- All children with cancer will experience pain. This experience may be related to the disease or its treatment.
- Poor pain management has a significant impact on the quality of life, the well-being of the child and family (physical and emotional), and daily functioning.

Incidence

- The main cause of pain in children diagnosed and undergoing therapy for cancer is treatment-related pain.
- Approximately 80 % of children with cancer suffer significantly at end of life, yet less than 30 % of these children are treated successfully.

Etiology

- Tumor related: Due to infiltration, obstruction of, or injury to the tissues, organs, and/or nerves:
  ○ Bone fractures.
  ○ Chest or pleuritic pain.
  ○ Brain: Headaches, intracranial pressure.
  ○ Abdomen/pelvis: Lumbosacral plexus compression, back pain, sciatica.
- Treatment related:
  ○ Chemotherapy: Vincristine (neuropathic).
  ○ Surgery/procedural: Incisions; infection; trauma; lumbar punctures; venipunctures, intravenous access procedures; bone marrow aspirates/biopsies.

Table 13-1 Common types and causes of pain in pediatric oncology.

Nociceptive Pain:	Neuropathic Pain
• Stimuli produced by peripheral nerve endings that are triggered in response to tissue or organ damage • Bone disease pain arises from the irritation and distension of pain receptors in the periosteum and endosteum • Responsive to nonopioid and opioid	• Stimuli produced by the altered excitability of the central or peripheral nerve as a result of nerve infiltration, injury, compression, and/or destruction • Complex and difficult to completely control • Sensation may continue even after the original injury has healed • Hyperalgesia and/or allodynia often present • Persistent pain relatively not responsive to typical opioid therapy • "Burning," "stabbing," "shooting," "tingling"

Somatic	Visceral	Centrally Generated	Peripherally Generated
• Arises from bone, joint, muscle, skin, or connective tissue • "Achy," "sharp," "throbbing"	• Organ involvement and nociceptors activated by the distention or inflammation of visceral organs • Metabolic alteration • Obstruction of hollow viscous, which causes intermittent cramping and poorly localized pain	• *Differentiation pain:* injury to either the peripheral or central nervous system • Burning below the level of the spinal cord lesion reflects injury to the CNS • *Sympathetically maintained pain:* dysregulation of the autonomic nervous system	• *Polyneuropathies* involves the distribution of many peripheral nerves • *Mononeuropathies* related to known peripheral nerve injury. • Sock-and-glove pain: abnormal sensation of the feet and hands "numbness" or "pins and needles"

○ Radiation: Burns; fibrosis or scarring to connective and nerve tissues.

○ Mucositis: Somatic pain related to the destruction of the mucosal lining from systemic (chemotherapy) and local (radiation) effects of cancer therapy.

○ Graft-versus-host disease.

Assessment: The 5th Vital Sign

- Patient and family-centered approach: Ensure the health and well-being of the patient and their family by:
  ○ Recognizing them as important partners in the assessment, planning, delivery, and evaluation of health care.
  ○ Considering issues related to culture, values, beliefs, knowledge, perspectives, and choices.
- Assess and reassess patients with acute and chronic pain at regular intervals depending on the etiology, degree, and control of/over the pain (e.g., every shift; hourly; every 15 minutes). This should also occur after:
  ○ The initiation of treatment.
  ○ Each new report of pain.
  ○ Any uncomfortable/painful intervention.
- Use validated pain assessment tools based on the child's physiological, cognitive, and emotional development such as:
  ○ Premature Infant Pain Profile (PIPP): Preterm and full-term neonates.
  ○ FLACC tool: 2 months to 7 years; nonverbal older and/or cognitively impaired.
  ○ Pain word scale (none, a little, medium, a lot) for 3–7 years.

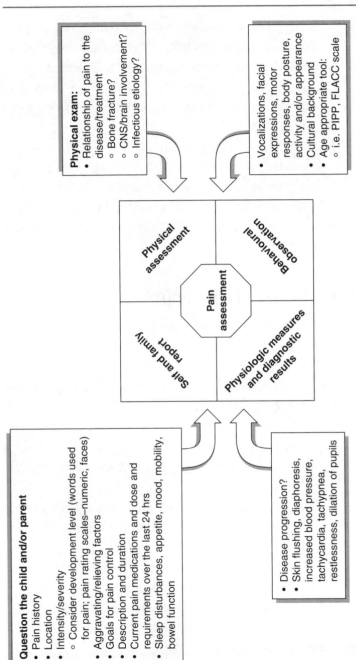

Physical exam:
- Relationship of pain to the disease/treatment
  - Bone fracture?
  - CNS/brain involvement?
  - Infectious etiology?

- Vocalizations, facial expressions, motor responses, body posture, activity and/or appearance
- Cultural background
- Age appropriate tool:
  - i.e. PIPP, FLACC scale

Question the child and/or parent
- Pain history
- Location
- Intensity/severity
  - Consider development level (words used for pain; pain rating scales—numeric, faces)
- Aggravating/relieving factors
- Goals for pain control
- Description and duration
- Current pain medications and dose and requirements over the last 24 hrs
- Sleep disturbances, appetite, mood, mobility, bowel function

- Disease progression?
- Skin flushing, diaphoresis, increased blood pressure, tachycardia, tachypnea, restlessness, dilation of pupils

Physical assessment

Behavioural observation

Pain assessment

Self and family report

Physiologic measures and diagnostic results

Figure 13-1   Components of a comprehensive pain assessment.

○ Faces Pain Scale—Revised (FPS-R) for 5–12 years.

○ Noncommunicating Children's Pain Checklist (NCCPC-R): 3–18 years who are unable to speak because of cognitive impairments or disabilities, and may experience pain in hospital, at home, or in long-term care setting.

○ Noncommunicating Children's Pain Checklist—*Postoperative* version (NCCPC-PV) for 3–18 years who are unable to speak because of cognitive impairments or disabilities for postop or procedural pain in hospital.

○ Numerical Rating Scale (NRS): 0–10 for 7 years and older.

Barriers to Good Pain Control

• Lack of knowledge in pharmacological and nonpharmacological interventions associated with pain control.

• Myths and misconceptions regarding the use of opioids (When appropriately administered):

○ Addiction is very rare in children being treated for pain.

○ Addiction is the voluntary psychological dependency on a drug.

○ Tolerance is the involuntary physiological adaptation to a drug in which higher doses are required to control the desired symptom.

○ Dependence is the involuntary physiological effect related to the abrupt discontinuation of an opioid.

○ Risks or dangers regarding opioid use are not greater than that of adults, and there is *no greater* risk of respiratory depression.

• Poor assessment of pain.

Management

- The basic principle of pain management is the full utilization of the 3 *P*s concept: physical, psychological, pharmacological:
  - Physical and psychological: Techniques to manage pain should be an integral part of all pain management strategies. Some of these techniques are radiation therapy, warm or cold compresses, baths, massage, distraction, deep breathing, muscle relaxation, positioning, swaddling, guided imagery, and music, clown, art, and play therapy.
  - Pharmacological intervention using the principles of balanced analgesia: This includes prescribing by *the ladder*, around *the clock*, by *mouth* where possible, and tailored to the *child's* need(s). Establish etiology of the pain when possible.
- Use a patient- and family-centered approach that consciously adopts the patient's perspective about issues that matter.
- Goals of pain management are to prevent and relieve pain and to preserve and restore the quality of life of the patient and his or her family, while minimizing treatment side effects.
- Be proactive:
  - Discussions about pain and pain control should not be left to the last minute.
  - Patients and families should be prepared to deal with painful conditions early in the disease cycle.
  - Discuss available and practical pain management options and concepts with the patient and family such as the principles of pain management; setting treatment goals, and monitoring outcomes (efficacy, tolerance, and side effects).

○ Consider:

- Adding medical and nonmedical interventions to control/prevent side effects from opioids and other adjunctive treatments (stool softeners and stimulants, antiemetics).

- An opioid rotation: Use when the escalating opioid dose is not achieving the desired pain control and resulting in intolerable or uncontrolled side effects. Start at, or just below, the morphine equivalence dose (e.g., rotating from morphine to hydromorphone due to severe itching).

- Use oral long-acting opioids in persistent but controlled pain, in addition to short acting opioids to control breakthrough pain.

- Use an opioid infusion in moderate to severe pain when trying to aggressively control pain or when oral route not an option (e.g., mucositis):
  □ Hourly rate (HR) = the sum of the patient's opioid need (ON) in last 24 h, *plus:*
  □ An additional 10–25% of the patients previous opioid needs (B).
  □ HR = (ON + B)/24.

- An opioid rescue = 10–25% of daily opioid need available for breakthrough pain as needed (PRN).

- For refractory pain, consider:
  □ Neuropathic pain as the potential etiology.
  □ Adding adjunctive treatment.
  □ Consulting pain specialists.

- Other important issues to consider:
  □ Respiratory depression is a rare side effect of opioids when the dose is monitored and titrated appropriately.

Text continued on page 218

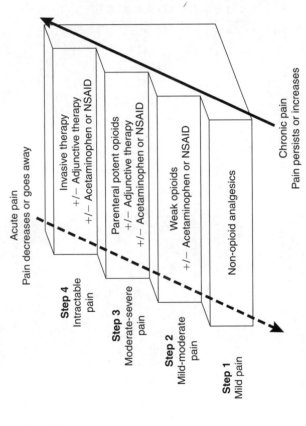

Figure 13-2 Therapeutic ladder for pain management.

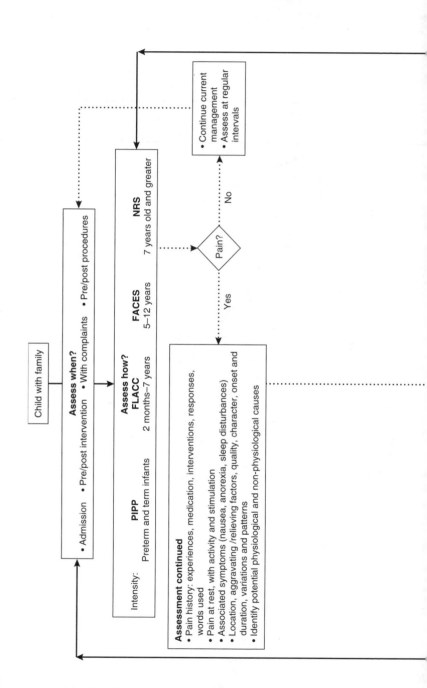

Child with family

Assess when?
• Admission • Pre/post intervention • Pre/post procedures • With complaints

Assess how?

PIPP	**FLACC**	**FACES**	**NRS**
Preterm and term infants	2 months–7 years	5–12 years	7 years old and greater

Intensity:

Pain?
Yes
No

• Continue current management
• Assess at regular intervals

Assessment continued
• Pain history: experiences, medication, interventions, responses, words used
• Pain at rest, with activity and stimulation
• Associated symptoms (nausea, anorexia, sleep disturbances)
• Location, aggravating /relieving factors, quality, character, onset and duration, variations and patterns
• Identify potential physiological and non-physiological causes

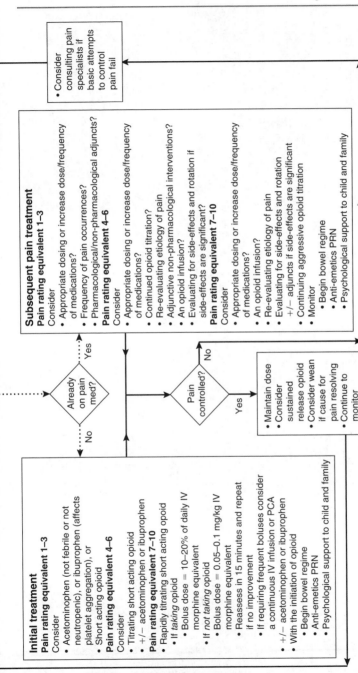

Initial treatment

Pain rating equivalent 1–3

Consider

- Acetominophen (not febrile or not neutropenic), or ibuprophen (affects platelet aggregation), or
- Short acting opioid

Pain rating equivalent 4–6

Consider

- Titrating short acting opioid
- +/– acetominophen or ibuprophen

Pain rating equivalent 7–10

Rapidly titrating short acting opioid

- If *taking* opioid
  - Bolus dose = 10–20% of daily IV morphine equivalent
- If *not taking* opioid
  - Bolus dose = 0.05–0.1 mg/kg IV morphine equivalent
- Reassess in 15 minutes and repeat if no improvement
- If requiring frequent boluses consider a continuous IV infusion or PCA
- +/– acetominophen or ibuprophen
- With the initiation of opioid
  - Begin bowel regime
  - Anti-emetics PRN
  - Psychological support to child and family

Already on pain med? No / Yes

Pain controlled? No / Yes

- Maintain dose
- Consider sustained release opioid
- Consider wean if cause for pain resolving
- Continue to monitor

Subsequent pain treatment

Pain rating equivalent 1–3

Consider

- Appropriate dosing or increase dose/frequency of medications?
- Frequency of pain occurrences?
- Pharmacological/non-pharmacological adjuncts?

Pain rating equivalent 4–6

Consider

- Appropriate dosing or increase dose/frequency of medications?
- Continued opioid titration?
- Re-evaluating etiology of pain
- Adjunctive non-pharmacological interventions?
- An opioid infusion?
- Evaluating for side-effects and rotation if side-effects are significant?

Pain rating equivalent 7–10

Consider

- Appropriate dosing or increase dose/frequency of medications?
- An opioid infusion?
- Re-evaluating etiology of pain
- Evaluating for side-effects and rotation +/– adjuncts if side-effects are significant
- Continuing aggressive opioid titration
- Monitor
  - Begin bowel regime
  - Anti-emetics PRN
  - Psychological support to child and family

- Consider consulting pain specialists if basic attempts to control pain fail

Figure 13-3 Algorithm for pain assessment and management.

Table 13-2 Pharmacological pain intervention according to the quality of pain.

Quality	Drug	Dosing	Dose Limits	Assess	Considerations
Mild	Acetaminophen	10–15 mg/kg PO q 4 h	75 mg/kg/day or 4 g/day, whichever is less. Children >12 y	Ease of administration schedule	In adjunctive therapy, can reduce opioid dose by 30–35%.
	NSAIDS (Cox inhibitors) Ibuprophen	5–10 mg/kg PO q 6–8 h	40 mg/kg/day or 2400 mg/day	Dosing Adherence Need to change to different NSAID if ineffective or unacceptable side effects	Decrease opioid side effects May mask fevers and affect platelet aggregation (NSAIDS)
	Ketorolac (Cox-2 Inhibitor)	0.5 mg/kg IV q 6–8 h	15 mg max/dose for 24–48 h	Multidimensional assessment of pain	Ketorolac—use for 24–48 h then change to ibuprofen or diclofenac
	Celebrex	200–400 mg PO q 8 h	No dosing information for children < 18 y	Effectiveness of medication	
	Diclofenac	1 mg/kg 8–12 h	50 mg/dose or 3 mg/kg/day		
Moderate	Codeine	1 mg/kg PO q 4 h	5 mg/dose q 4–6 h		Caucasians (6–10%), Asians (2%), and the Arabs (1%) have poorly functioning cytochrome P450 enzyme CYP2D6, thereby limiting the metabolism and effectiveness of this drug
	Oxycodone	Instant release: 0.05–0.15 mg/kg/dose q 4–6 h Sustained release: 10 mg q 12 h—if taking > 20 mg/day			
	Morphine sulphate (short acting)	0.15 mg/kg/dose PO q 4 h PRN			

			Up to 2 % will have multiple copies of the enzyme CYP2D6; therefore, it metabolizes codeine to morphine faster and increases the risk of toxicity.
			Do not crush sustained relief meds.
			Any side effects?
			When starting *any opioid*: Start stool softeners daily with stimulant PRN.
Severe	Morphine sulphate	2 mg/dose	Do not crush sustained relief meds
		Rescue	Ensure appropriate rescue dosing
		0.3 mg/kg/dose PO q 4 h PRN	No ceiling effect, but if experiencing intolerable side effects consider a dose equivalent opioid rotation +/− adjunctive therapy
		0.05–0.1 mg/kg IV q2–4 PRN	
		Continuous infusion:	
		10–40 mcg/kg/h	
		(Prep: ½ × weight in kg in mg of morphine in 50 nl NS, 1 ml/h = 10 mcg/kg/h	
		Start @ 2 ml/h	

Consider dose equivalent sustained relief such as (ms-contin, m-eslon) when pain adequately managed parentally

For opioid infusions:

Titrate as necessary

(continued)

Table 13-2 (continued).

Quality	Drug	Dosing	Dose Limits	Assess	Considerations
Severe (continued)	Hydromorphone	*Rescue:* 0.06 mg/kg PO q 3–4 h 0.01–02 mg/kg IV q 3–4 h *Continuous Infusion:* 4–6 mcg/kg/h (Prep: 0.1 × wt in kg in mg hydromorphone in 50 mls NS, 1 ml/h + 2 mcg/kg/h, start @ 2 ml/h	0.5 mg/dose		*With any opioids:* Start antiemetics PRN. Stool softeners daily with stimulant PRN. Consider PCA pump if: Used in eligible children > 6 yr (or in developmentally appropriate children) If so, consult the acute pain service
	Fentanyl	*Rescue:* Start 0.5–2.0 mcg/kg/dose *Continuous Infusion:* 0.5–1 mcg/kg/h (Prep: 50 × wt in kg in mcg fentanyl in 50 ml NS: 1 ml/h = 1 mcg/kg/h)Start @ 0.5 ml/h *Transdermal patch*	50 mcg/dose		Tapering opioids after long use: Decrease by approx 10–20% every day—every other day (slower if there are signs of withdrawal) May require consultation with palliative care and/or pain specialists

				Consider the fentanyl patch in a patient who: Cannot tolerate oral opioid; Has poor veins Does not want an IV Patch duration = 72 h Contraindicated in: Infants or small children when dose is less than the smallest patch (patches should not be cut or altered in any way) Febrile child due to risk of increased transdermal drug absorption
Intractable	**Neuropathic Interventions** Antiepileptic Gabapentin (Gold Standard)	Day 1: 5 mg/kg PO q h Day 2: BID Day 3: TID Titrate to effect by 100 mg q 2 days Usual starting dose 100 mg	Max starting dose: 100 mg	Sedating effects	Consider: Adequate dosing (infusion and/or rescue dosing)? Need for other adjunctive therapy? Pain of neuropathic origin (burning, numbness, or paresthesia, and hypersensitive) No drug levels
	Tricyclic antidepressants Amytriptyline	0.2–0.5 mg/kg PO q h	Max adult dose 900 mg TID	Sedating effects TDM levels	
	Anticonvulsants Carbamazepine	Titrate by 0.25 mg/kg every 5–7 days as required	Max: 100 mg/dose Max: 1.6–2.4 g/day	Sedating effects TDM levels	

(continued)

Table 13-2 (continued).

Quality	Drug	Dosing	Dose Limits	Assess	Considerations
Intractable (continued)		Usual starting dose 10–25 mg < 6 y 2.5–5 mg PO BID Titrate to affect weekly by 20 mg/kg/day 6–12 y 5 mg/kg PO BID Titrate to affect weekly by 10 mg/kg/day > 12 y 200 mg BID Titrate to affect weekly by 200 mg/day			Analgesia within hrs to days No probable antidepressant effects Give at night Onset within hours
Other Adjuncts	Dexamethasone Clonidine *Ketamine* Sufentanyl Methadone	Dose dependent on clinical situations Cerebral edema 1–2 mg/kg load then 1–1.5/kg/day divided by q 6 h dosing Anti-inflammatory: 0.08–0.3 mg/kg/day divided by 6–12 h dosing 1–2 mcg/kg q 8 h			Side effects to consider: Edema, gastrointestinal irritation, mood swings, acne, hunger, inc. blood pressure Add: H2 blockers (ranitidine) or proton pump inhibitors (omeprazole)

Under the direction and observation of a palliative care and/or pain specialist

Intractable neuropathic pain

Monitor for potential increase in the hallucination or nightmares

Under the direction and observation of a methadone-licensed palliative care and/or pain specialist

NOTES:

SDL = Single dose limit

Table 13-3 Management of opioid-related side effects.

Side Effect	Pharmacological Intervention	Dosing	Nonpharmacological Intervention	Considerations
Constipation	Stool softener +/− Docusate	Oral < 3–10 y: 40 mg/day 3–6 y: 20–60 mg/day 6–12 y: 40–150 mg/day > 12 y: 50–400 mg/day May divide into o.d. or QID dosing Onset: 24–48 hrs Rectal < 6 y: 1 pediatric supp 1–2 × day > 6 y: 1 adult supp 1–2×/day Onset: 20–60 minutes	Fibrous diet Water Abdominal massage Exercise	Begin prophylactic regimen with a stool softener on a regular basis and a cathartic, lubricant, or stimulant PRN Add lubricants or stimulants if no relief Continue prophylactic regime once relieved Rectal route of drug administration is contraindicated in children who are neutropenic Dose limit: Citrate: 300 ml/dose Oxide: Usual adult dose 30–60 ml
	Cathartic Senna	4 m to 12 y: 4 mg/kg daily or may divide dose and give BID > 12 y: 15–30 mg o.d.–BID Onset: 8–12 h		
	Lubricant Lactulose	4 m to 12 y: 5–10 ml o.d.–TID		
	Stimulant Bisacodyl (oral or rectal)	> 12 y: 10–15 ml BID–TID Onset: 36–48 h		

	Magnesium	5 mg–10 mg PO o.d. Onset: 10–12 h (oral)	
	Magnesium citrate	20–60 min (rectal) 2–4 ml/kg/dose PO	
	Magnesium hydroxide	0.5 ml/kg/PO (33 mg elemental mg/ml) Onset: 0.5–3 h	
Opioid-induced sedation	Caffeine	2.5–5 mg q a.m. and early afternoon PRN	Caffeinated drinks Common side effect that is more distressing for parents than child
	Methylphenidate		If pain managed consider decreasing opioid dose by 10%. If pain increases consider adjunctive therapy If pain continues, reconsider starting at previous dose, reassure parents, and consider stimulant If no pain, continue at this dose Potential indication for opioid rotation?

(continued)

Table 13-2 (continued).

Side Effect	Pharmacological Intervention	Dosing	Nonpharmacological Intervention	Considerations
Pruritis	**Antihistamine** Diphenhydramine Hydroxyzine Low-dose naloxone	1 mg/kg/dose PO/IV q 4–6 h 0.6 mg/kg/dose PO q 6 h 0.5–2 mcg/kg/h continuous infusion (Prep: 0.4 mg (1 ml) Naloxone in 39 ml NS, final concentration is 1 ml = 10 mcg Start @ 0.5 mcg/kg/h	Cold or warm compresses Oatmeal bath	Dose limit: Diphenhydramine: 50 mg/dose Hydroxyzine: 50 mg/dose
Nausea and vomiting	Ondansetron Granisetron Dimenhydrinate Lorazepam	0.1–0.15 mg/kg PO/IV q 8 h 10 mcg/kg q 12 h 1 mg/kg PO/IV q 6 h 0.025 mg/kg IV/PO/sl	Imagery, relaxation, deep slow breathing	Dose limit: Ondansetron: 8 mg/dose Granisetron: 1 mg/dose Dimenhydrinate: 50 mg/dose Lorazepam: 2 mg/dose
Urinary retention	Oxybutynin	< 5 y: 0.125 mg/kg/dose PO QID > 5 y: 5 mg/dose PO BID–TID	Warm compresses to bladder Turn faucet to a "trickle"	Assess bladder size Consider intermittent catheterization Potential indication for opioid rotation Rule out anatomical causes

- ■ Acetaminophen and NSAIDs should be prescribed with caution due to its antipyretic and antiplatelet effects, respectively.
- ■ Meperidine for analgesia is not recommended due to CNS effects from the accumulation of a toxic metabolite (normeperidine).
- Palliative and end-of-life pain: Management follows the same principles as above. In addition more techniques of controlling pain are utilized. This may include:
  - ○ Sedation, peripheral nerve blocks, epidural analgesia, spinal analgesia, plexus blocks, denervation techniques, intrathecal stimulation, ketamine infusion.
  - ○ May require consultation with the palliative care team and/or pain specialists.

References

American Pain Society. *Guideline for the Management of Cancer Pain in Adults and Children*. Glenview, IL: American Pain Society; 2005.

Ferrell B, Rhiner M, Shapiro B, Dierkes M. The experience of pediatric cancer pain, part II: the management of pain, *J Pediatr Nurs*. 1994;9(6): 368–379.

Hockenberry-Eaton M, Barrera P, Brown M, Bottomley S, O'Neil J. *Pain Management in Children with Cancer*. Houston, TX: Texas Cancer Council; 1999. http://www.childcancerpain.org/contents/childpainmgmt.pdf. Accessed 2008-07-22.

Hospital for Sick Children. *SickKids Drug Handbook and Formulary 2006–2007*. Toronto, Canada: Hospital for Sick Children; 2006.

Wolfe J, Grier H, Klar N, et al. Symptoms and suffering at the end of life in children with cancer. *N Engl J Med*. 2000;342(5):326–333.

World Health Organization. *Cancer pain relief and palliative care in children*. Geneva, Switzerland: World Health Organization; 1998.

chapter 14

Psychiatric Issues

Claire De Souza and Oussama Abla

Outline

- Introduction
- Common Psychiatric Presentations
- Pharmacologic Treatment
- Challenging Parents
- Clinician Well-Being

Introduction

Psychiatric Presentations in Pediatric Oncology Patients

- Are common and may be due to:
  - Medication/withdrawal or organic etiology; delirium.
  - Cognitive problems, sensory problems, pain.
  - Adjustment disorder, mood disorder, anxiety disorder, psychotic disorder.
- May present as treatment refusal or nonadherence.

- Multiple losses for patient, including health, notion of immortality, meaning, control, predictability, normality, autonomy, relationships, security, potential, productivity, finances.
- Losses may result in powerlessness, hopelessness, uncertainty, loneliness, isolation, grief.

Impact of Illness by Developmental Stage

Preschooler: Age 3–5 Years

- Child may view illness, treatment, procedures as punishment for bad behavior.
- Normal task to separate from parents and explore environment may be affected through parental overprotection and separation from parent with hospitalization.

School-Aged Child: Age 6–12 Years

- Child has some capacity to understand illness and treatment, but may view illness as punishment for bad behavior or due to contact with germs.
- Child may fear harm to body, worry about death.
- Normal task to gain a sense of mastery via academic, physical, and social challenges may be affected due to illness → school absenteeism, parental overprotection, and fewer social interactions resulting in alienation from peers.

Adolescent: Age 13–19 Years

- Greater understanding of illness and mind-body connection. Recurrence may be seen as punishment; survival may be viewed with guilt or imply special purpose.
- Normal task to focus on identity, appearance, growth, autonomy, and relationships may be affected with fears of disfigurement and death, loss of a sense of invincibility, alienation from peers, academic disruptions with

concern for future achievement, and loss of independence. Control may be sought through nonadherence.

Healthcare Provider Must Assess the Impact of Illness and Treatment on the Child/Adolescent and Family

- Developmental age, stage of the family, culture, psychiatric history.
- Family's understanding of illness, treatment, side effects; impact of illness and treatment on family (interpret case history psychosocially); anticipated sources of stress; family's experience of illness in others (family, friends); history of loss and coping; coping, supports.

Common Psychiatric Presentations

Delirium (Encephalopathy, Acute Confusional State)

Clinical Presentation

- Disturbance of consciousness, impaired alertness.
- Reduced ability to focus, sustain, or shift attention; distractible.
- Cognitive changes (even during lucid times)—"Confused," disoriented (time, place), poor short-term memory (immediate, recent, procedural), language disturbance (dysarthria, dysnomia, aphasia, dysgraphia), constructional apraxia, executive dysfunction (problems with information processing, reasoning, problem solving, anticipating consequences, abstraction).
- Perceptual changes, delusional symptoms: "In a dream," misinterpretations, misidentification, illusions, hallucinations (visual, tactile, etc.), paranoia.
- Psychomotor disturbance: Agitation, slowing.
- Affect: Irritable, angry, anxious, fearful, sad, euphoric; labile, rapid changes.

- Speech: Incoherent, mumbling, rambling, mute.
- Thought form: Disorganized, tangential, loosening of associations.
- Sleep disturbance: "Sundowning," daytime sleepiness, night time agitation.
- Neurological signs: Tremor, change in reflexes and tone, myoclonus, asterixis.

Subtypes

- Hyperactive: Hyperalert, agitated, combative, loud/fast speech, psychotic.
- Hypoactive: Somnolent, confused, slowed down, decreased speech, sad affect.
- Mixed.

Clinical Course

- Prodrome—hours to days before: Anxious, irritable, distractible, withdrawn, restless, disturbed sleep (nightmares), illusions, hallucinations.
- Develops over a short period of time (hours to days), fluctuates over the day.
- Lasts less than 1 week to over 2 months, average 10–12 days.
- May have perceptual, motor changes for weeks; limited recall of negative aspects.
- Risk of stupor, coma, death.

Etiology

Due to medical condition and/or substance/medication/toxin.

- Examples:
  - Medications:
    - Cytarabine, bleomycin, carmustine, cisplatin, dacarbazine, fludarabine, 5-FU, interferon, inter-

leukin, ifosfamide, L-asparaginase, methotrexate, prednisone, procarbazine, tamoxifen, vinblastine, vincristine.

- Acyclovir, ganciclovir, isoniazid, rifampin, amphoterin B, ciprofloxacin, metronidazole.
- Antihistamines, steroids, naproxen, ibuprofen, opiates, metoclopramide, anticonvulsants.
- Antiarrhythmics, sympathomimetics, antihypertensives.
- Antidepressants, antipsychotics, benzodiazepines, benztropine.

Note: drug interactions; withdrawal (opiods, benzodiazepines)

○ Infection:
- Encephalitis, meningitis, sepsis, pneumonia, urinary tract infection, HIV, syphilis.

○ Neoplastic:
- Tumor, paraneoplastic syndrome.

○ CNS:
- Seizures, hydrocephalus, hemorrhage, stroke, tumour, vasculitis, radiation.

○ Metabolic/endocrine:
- Fluid/electrolyte, acid/base, hyper/hypoglycemia, renal/liver failure, thyroid disease, hyper/hypo-adrenocorticism, hyperparathyroidism.

○ Vascular:
- Arrhythmia, stroke, hypertensive encephalopathy, shock, hypotension.

○ Hypoxia:
- Anemia, cardiac/pulmonary failure, pulmonary embolus.

○ Nutritional deficiency:
- Thiamine, B_{12}, folate, niacin.

○ Heavy metals/toxins:
  ■ Lead, manganese, mercury, pesticides.
○ Trauma:
  ■ Closed head injury, burns.
○ Other:
  ■ Porphyria.

Assessment

- Chart review; history/physical including neurological, vital signs (VS), O_2 sat.
- Mini-Mental State Examination (MMSE): orientation, attention, recall, following commands.
- Investigations to consider:
  ○ Blood: CBC, electrolytes, glucose, BUN, creatinine, AST/ALT/ALP, bilirubin, albumin, Ca^{2+}/Mg^{2+}/PO_{4-}, arterial blood gases (ABGs), TSH, B_{12}, RBC folate, osmolality, ESR, ANA, LE prep, cortisol, NH_{4+}, heavy metal screen, HIV, VDRL, blood culture.
  ○ Urine: Urinalysis, drug screen, drug levels, urinary porphyrins.
  ○ Lumbar puncture.
  ○ ECG, EEG (global slowing); imaging: CXR, CT +/− MRI, MRA.

Management

- Treat underlying cause; avoid or minimize anticholinergics and narcotics.
- Monitor VS, O_2 sat, ins/outs, mood, behavior, suicidal/homicidal ideation, cognition, psychosis, and sleep.
- Supportive measures: Constant observation due to risk of falls, wandering, suicidal ideation (SI), homicidal ideation (HI):
  ○ Chemical restraints for agitation.

○ Education, support to patient and family; family to reassure patient.

- Environmental measures: Well-lit private room: lights on during day, turned down at night; minimize noise/stimulation; familiar items (photos, toys); familiar people; orienting cues: clock, calendar.
- Psychiatry consult.
- Medications: low-dose atypical antipsychotics (risperidone) or haloperidol. Avoid benzodiazepines due to risk of confusion, sedation, paradoxical agitation, respiratory depression; use benzodiazepines if sedative withdrawal.

Depression

Clinical Presentation

- Mood: Depressed, irritable, bored, angry, discouraged; ± anxious.
- Changes in sleep, appetite, weight, energy.
- Psychosomatic complaints—medically unexplained symptoms:
  ○ Headaches, abdominal pain, fatigue, weakness, GI problems, etc.
  ○ Mood improves with reduced pain; low mood exacerbates pain.
- Cognitive: Hopeless, helpless, worthless, SI, inattentive, guilt ± psychosis.
- Behavioural: Agitated or slowed down:
  ○ Preschooler: Tantrums, regression.
  ○ Child/adolescent: Disruptive behaviour, treatment refusal, nonadherence.
- Interpersonal: Decreased interest, withdrawal.

Etiology

- Examples:
  - Medications:
    - Amphoterin B, beta blockers, clonidine, corticosteroids, vincristine, cyclosporine, interferon, L-asparaginase, methadone, contraceptives, oxycodone, procarbazine, procainamide, tacrolimus, vinblastine, vincristine.
  - Infections:
    - Encephalitis, influenza, mononucleosis, pneumonia, subacute bacterial endocarditis, hepatitis, AIDS, tuberculosis, syphilis.
  - Endocrine/metabolic:
    - Diabetes, Cushing's, Addison's, hyper/hypothyroidism, hyper/hypoparathyroidism, hyper/hypokalemia, hyponatremia, hypophosphatemia.
  - Malignancy:
    - Tumors of the CNS, lung, pancreas; paraneoplastic.
  - CNS:
    - Epilepsy, postconcussion syndrome, stroke, sleep apnea, subarachnoid hemorrhage.
  - Nutritional:
    - Failure to thrive; vitamin D, B_{12}, folate deficiency.
  - Renal:
    - Uremia, hemodialysis.
  - Other:
    - Chronic pain, anemia.

Assessment

- History, physical, VS, O_2 sat.
- Investigations to consider:
  - CBC, electrolytes, glucose, renal, LFTs, TSH, ABGs, cortisol, albumin, Ca^{2+}/PO_{4-}, B_{12}, RBC folate, urinalysis, drug screen; ECG, EEG; CXR; CT/MRI; LP.

Differential Diagnosis

- Mood disorder due to medical condition; delirium; substance induced mood disorder.
- Major depressive disorder: Often has past psychiatric history and family history.
- Adjustment disorder with depressed mood: Milder, responds to distraction.
- Bereavement: Terminal stage, anticipatory grief.
- Bipolar disorder.

Management

- Monitor mood, behavior, sleep, suicidal ideation, and physical complaints.
- Supportive: Child Life can create a schedule of activities; teacher; playroom:
  - Friends, volunteers, access to Internet, chaplaincy; music therapy.
  - Education: "depression is common and treatable."
- Environmental: Bright room, familiar toys.
- Consultation: Social work, psychology, psychiatry for psychotherapy.
- Medications: In moderate-severe depression, minimum 9–12 mo; taper if stopping:
  - SSRIs—First-line if no bipolar disorder.

Suicidal Ideation (SI)

Assessment

Meet with child/teen and parent:

- "Some people get so overwhelmed and depressed that they think about hurting themselves or wish they were dead. Have you ever felt/been feeling this badly?"

- Assess how recent, intense, frequent, and specific the thoughts and feelings are; passive wish to be dead vs. intent and plan to harm or kill self; seriousness of plan, lethality; impulsivity, substance use, previous self-harm/suicide attempts (and seriousness), access to guns, pills, sharps; supervision, supports.

Management

- Monitor: Close follow-up; fill out form 1 (application by a physician for a psychiatric assessment to take place in hospital ER or ward, which lasts up to 72 hrs) if unwilling to stay in hospital and at risk:
  - Constant observation if moderate to high risk: Child and youth worker, security, or parent.
- Supportive measures: Discuss with child/adolescent and parents:
  - Address stressors that increase suicidal ideation (e.g., somatic complaints, pain).
  - Safety planning: Agreement not to self-harm, attempt suicide; outline coping strategies (relaxation, distraction, activities, supports, staff).
- Environmental: Safety of room—remove sharps, medications; inform team.
- Psychiatry consult—suicide risk assessment and treatment.

Mania/Hypomania

Clinical Presentation

- Mood: Irritable, angry, elated; ± anxious.
- Physical: Decreased need for sleep (also a trigger), increased energy and sex drive.

- Cognitive: Grandiose, distractible, racing thoughts, poor judgment; ± psychosis.
- Behavior: Agitated; pressured speech; increase in pleasurable, risky activities.
- *Note:* Mixed states (depression + mania during the same episode) are common in teens.

Etiology

- Examples:
  - Medications:
    - Antidepressants, bronchodilators, captopril, carbamazepine, cimetidine, corticosteroids, decongestants, lorazepam, methlyphenidate, metoclopramide, procarbazine, thyroid medications.
  - Endocrine/metabolic:
    - Cushing's, hyper/hypothyroidism, hypocalcemia.
  - CNS:
    - Epilepsy, multiple sclerosis, postconcussion, stroke, Wilson's.
  - Infectious:
    - Encephalitis, influenza, mononucleosis, AIDS, syphilis.
  - Heme-Onc:
    - Gliomas, meningiomas, thalamic, carcinoid; anemia.
  - Renal:
    - Uremia, hemodialysis.
  - Nutritional:
    - Niacin deficiency, vitamin B_{12} deficiency.

Assessment

- History, physical exam including neurological, VS, O_2 sat
- Investigations to consider:
  - CBC, electrolytes, renal, LFTs, Ca^{2+}, cortisol, B_{12}, TSH, ABGs, drug screen, ECG.

Differential Diagnosis

- Mood disorder due to medical condition; delirium; substance induced mood disorder.
- Bipolar disorder.
- ADHD.

Management

- Monitor mood, sleep, behavior, psychosis, and suicidal ideation.
- Supportive measures: Constant observation.
- Environmental measures: Low stimulation, own room; sleep restoration is key.
- Psychiatry consult.
- Medications: Atypical antipsychotic +/− mood stabilizer, stop antidepressant.

Anxiety

Clinical Presentation

- Mood: Scared, anxious; moody; psychosomatic complaints.
- Physical: Hyperventilation, palpitations, nausea, tense muscles, dizziness.
- Cognitive: "Something bad is going to happen" and "I can't cope."
- Behavior: Avoidance; agitation ± nonadherence or treatment refusal.

Etiology

- Examples:
  - Medications:
    - Anti-asthmatics, anticholinergics, antidepressants, antiemetics (metoclopromide), antihistamines, an-

tipsychotics, cold medications, sympathomimetics, steroids, metronidazole, thyroid medications, withdrawal (opiate, steroid, ativan).

○ Endocrine/metabolics:
  ■ Hyper/hypothyroid, hypoglycemia, diabetes, hyperkalemia, hyper/hypocalcemia, hypomagnesemia, hypophosphatemia, carcinoid syndrome.

○ CNS:
  ■ Migraine, seizure, encephalopathy, vertigo, stroke, postconcussive syndrome.

○ CVS:
  ■ Arrhythmia, CHF, hypovolemia, valvular disease.

○ Respiratory:
  ■ Asthma, pulmonary edema, pneumothorax, pulmonary embolism, hypoxia.

○ Oncology:
  ■ Brain, pancreas, thyroid, parathyroid, adrenocorticotropic, pheochromocytoma.

○ Rheumatology:
  ■ SLE.

○ Toxin/substance:
  ■ Lead, caffeine.

○ Other:
  ■ Porphyria, anaphylaxis, hyperthermia, uncontrolled pain.

Assessment

• History, physical exam, VS, O_2 sat.
• Investigations to consider:
  ○ CBC, electrolytes, glucose, BUN, creatinine, LFTs, Ca^{2+}, Mg^{2+}, PO_{4-}, cortisol, TSH, ABGs, urinalysis, drug screen; CXR, ECG, cardiac monitoring, CT/MRI, EEG, LP.

Differential Diagnosis

- Anxiety due to medical condition; delirium; substance induced/withdrawal.
- Primary anxiety disorder:
  - Generalized anxiety disorder—Multiple worries (family, school, peers, activities, future, world) plus fatigue, insomnia, inattention, muscle tension.
  - Panic disorder—Sense of impending doom, physical symptoms.
  - Specific phobia—Situational, needle, etc., with avoidance behavior.
  - Obsessive compulsive disorder—Repetitive or ritualized behavior.
  - Acute stress disorder, post-traumatic stress disorder—Fearful traumatic event plus reexperiencing, dissociation, hyperarousal, avoidance.
  - Separation anxiety disorder—Worry about being separated from parent.
- Adjustment disorder with anxious mood.
- ADHD, learning disability, mood disorder, psychotic disorder, somatoform disorder, eating disorder, autism spectrum disorder.

Management

- Monitor mood, sleep, behavior, pain, and physical complaints.
- Supportive measures: Child Life, music therapy; chaplaincy.
- Environmental measures: Structured day: routine/schedule, preparation.
- Consultation: Social work, psychology, psychiatry for psychotherapy.
- Medications: Short-term only (procedure): Lorazepam; moderate-severe: SSRI.

- Cognitive behavioural approach (CBT):
  - Ratings (scale 1–10), visual analogues: Symptoms, functional status.
  - Cognitive restructuring: Correcting misconceptions (regarding diagnosis, treatment), evidence for/against? Best, worst, most realistic outcome? Positive self-talk.
  - Behavioural strategies:
    - Relaxation strategies:
      - Deep breathing: "In through nose × few seconds, pause × few seconds, out through mouth × few seconds, pause . . ."
      - Progressive muscle relaxation: "Starting with feet → head: tense each muscle group × few seconds then relax × few seconds . . ."
    - Create and post a schedule of activities, nursing care: to prepare.
    - Distraction: Toys, music, counting, videogames.
    - Procedures: Preparation, modeling, desensitization; offer choices.
    - Diary/graph of symptoms—post patient's progress on wall.
    - Use of rewards for coping.

Pharmacologic Treatment

Note: Keep in mind cytochrome P_{450} drug interactions.

Antidepressants (Involve Psychiatry)

- Principles: Start low, go slow; caution if history of hypomania or family history of bipolar disorder.
- Types: Citalopram, sertraline, fluoxetine; off-label.
- Indications: (1) Anxiety improves in 1–2 wks; (2) depression: sleep, energy, appetite improve in 2–3 wks → mood, cognition improve in 4–6 wks.

- Some evidence that medications work: benefits > risks; off-label use.
- Possible side effects: For 2 weeks after starting or with dose increase: nausea, stomach upset, headache, insomnia, dizziness; risk of platelet dysfunction.
- Discontinuation syndrome: Headaches, sleep problems, flu-like reaction, GI, anxiety, irritability with stopping suddenly.
- Health Canada and FDA warning: Small risk of agitation, disinhibition, akathisia (restlessness), hypomania, aggression, anxiety, insomnia, SI, self-harm behavior; therefore, need for monitoring: q 1–2 wks when starting/dose increase:
  ○ Rationale for warning: Activation effect, side effects, untreated symptoms/worsening mood, misdiagnosed/ hypomania.
- Serotonin syndrome: Nausea, diarrhea, dizziness, tachycardia, tachypnea, hypertension, fever, increased tone with twitching, tremor, hyperreflexia, myoclonus, unsteady gait, disorientation, agitation, restlessness, excitation, seizures, rhabdomyolysis, delirium, coma; rapid progression within 24 h:
  ○ Management: Stop SSRI, supportive care, decrease BP, cyproheptadine.
  ○ Risk with SSRIs, fentanyl, ondansetron, metoclopramide.

Antipsychotics (Involve Psychiatry)

- Types: Atypical (new) antipsychotics such as risperidone, olanzapine. Typical (old) antipsychotics are haloperidol (more extrapyramidal side effects [EPS]); chlorpromazine (less EPS, more anticholinergic).
- Principles: Start low, go slow; reassess daily.

- Some indications: Psychosis, aggression, agitation, delirium; off-label.
- Dosing depends on indication:
  - Risperidone 0.0625 mg–0.125 mg PO OD → BID (max 2 mg/24 h).
  - Olanzapine 1.25 mg–2.5 mg PO OD → BID (max 5–7.5 mg/24 h).
  - Haloperidol 0.25 mg–0.5 mg PO/IM/IV OD → BID (max 3 mg/24 h).
    - Give with lorazepam to minimize risk of EPS.
    - Use cardiac monitor for IV haloperidol.
- Side effects: Weight gain, CVS (increased HR, decreased BP), sedation, anticholingic (dry eyes, blurred vision, constipation, urinary retention).
- Risk:
  - EPS: (can occur with metoclopramide):
    - Dystonia (muscle spasm of tongue, neck, limbs, torso; oculogyric crisis; impaired breathing, etc.). Rx: Cogentin 1–2 mg PO/IM q 2 h PRN (max 4 mg/24 h).
    - Akathisia (restlessness; Rx: propanolol or lorazepam).
    - Neuroleptic malignant syndrome (NMS): Dysphagia, rigidity, tremor, altered consciousness, dysarthria, tachycardia, fever, tachypnea, autonomic instability, sweating, increased WBC, CPK, and myoglobinuria. Management: Stop antipsychotic; may give lorazepam, bromocryptine, or dantrolene.
    - Tardive dyskinesia.
  - Decreased seizure threshold, prolonged QTc interval, increased LFTs.
  - Increased prolactin, glucose/DM, lipid abnormalities, SIADH.
  - Agranulocytosis, neutropenia, aplastic anemia, thrombocytopenia.
- Baseline and monitor: CBC, glucose, LFTs, prolactin, lipid profile, ECG.

Anxiolytics (Short-Term Use Only (< 2 wks)

- Indications: Anxiety (e.g., pre-procedure), agitation, sleep, akathisia; not delirium.
- Side effects: Sedation, impaired mental speed, memory impairment; risk of confusion, disorientation, anticholinergic side effects, dizziness, respiratory depression, disinhibition (with young children; with delirium).
- Risk with prolonged use: Tolerance and withdrawal (dizziness, sweating, shaking, headache, nausea, insomnia, anxiety, depression, hypertension, muscle cramps, hallucinations, seizures).
- Dosing: Lorazepam 0.25 mg–0.5 mg PO/SL/IV q 4 h for anxiety, max 4 mg/24 h.

Sedatives

- Zopiclone: Short-term use (2 wks); dosing: 2.5 mg–7.5 mg qhs PRN for sleep.

Stimulants

- Low-dose methylphenidate (2.5 mg q a.m. & q lunch) for cancer-associated fatigue, malaise; potential side effects: nausea, decreased appetite, headache.

Challenging Parents

- What makes them challenging?
  - Complex, high needs patient; parental mental health problems.
  - Parents' reactions:
    - Feelings: Anger, rage, fear, uncertainty, shock, depression, substance use.

- ■ Behavior/actions: Overly involved, overly anxious, demanding, needing many medical opinions, idealizing ("best staff"), devaluing ("worst staff"), splitting ("good/bad" staff), aggressive, threatening, litigious; under-involved, withdrawn, nonadherent.
- Types of challenging families:
  - ○ "Dependent clingers" → desire to avoid: Limit set instead.
  - ○ "Entitled demanders" → desire to counterattack: Emphasize "partnership" that acknowledges entitlement to good medical care (but not unreasonable demands).
- Families "at risk" for developing problems:
  - ○ Single parent family; financial problems; cultural differences, preexisting family conflict (separated, divorced), medical/psychiatric problem in child/parent.

Team/Systems Approach

- Interprofessional meetings to debrief/plan:
  - ○ Review case and team members' concerns, process feelings, and problem solve.
  - ○ Involve various members as needed: Social work, psychiatry, patient advocate, ethics, risk management, administration, security (code white if violent/threatening), and child welfare as needed.
- Obtain 2nd opinions; obtain medico-legal advice as needed.
- Arrange point person, core care group; regular meetings with family for updates.
- Ensure concerns and plan are well documented and communicated to entire medical team.

Approach with Family

- Coordinate interprofessional meeting to gather all the information.
- Ensure sufficient time and privacy; meet with parents (separate from child).

Meeting with Parents (Without Child): Time Limited

- Allow parents to vent → reflect their distress.
- Prioritize issues: "We have _____ amount of time," "We would like to review _____," "What would you like to discuss?"
- Provide information in short, digestible chunks; avoid medical jargon/lecturing.
- Review their understanding and expectations of the diagnosis and treatment; correct misconceptions.
- Elicit thoughts and feelings: "What went through your mind when I said _____?," "What are you worried about?," "What do you think it means?," and "How are you feeling about what I've just said?"
- Validate their experience and feelings: "How has the diagnosis/treatment affected you?" and "How have you been feeling?" Use metaphors to reflect what the family is going through: like a rollercoaster, like waves, loss of control.
- Ask about coping: "How are you coping with the diagnosis/treatment? Sleeping? Eating? Taking breaks? Turning to supports?" Reinforce coping strategies; encourage connecting with supports and support groups.
- Tell them that they are part of the team with important roles: conveying information, providing support, decision making, medication management, etc.
- Increase their sense of control: Timetable, choices, anticipated sources of stress.

- Limit set aggression: "I understand that you are upset, but I cannot talk with you when you are yelling . . . I'll return when you calm down." Be equidistant to the exit, don't block the exit; if scared, leave the room or don't go in alone.
- Be aware of your own affect, behavior (body language, avoidance), cognition (thoughts about family, helplessness, repulsion, etc.).

Clinician Well-Being

Dealing with challenging patients and families puts additional stress on the healthcare provider, and steps must be taken to improve coping:

- Challenge distorted thinking to improve mood:
  - Challenge unrealistic expectations of self/others.
  - Limit setting, evidence for/against, best/worst/most realistic outcome.
  - Positive self-talk: I can do this, I'm making a difference etc; use of humor.
  - Keep a reflective journal; write thoughts down.
- Challenge behavior to improve mood:
  - Deep breathing, progressive muscle relaxation, meditation, etc.
  - Scheduled activities: Exercise, sports, vacation.
  - Adequate sleep, healthy diet.
- Interpersonal approaches: Regular debriefing of stressful cases, support network.

References

American Psychiatric Association. *Diagnostic and Statistical Manual of Mental Disorders*. 4th ed. Text revision. Washington, DC: American Psychiatric Association; 2000.

APA practice guidelines for the treatment of patients with delirium. *J Am Psychiatr Assoc*.1999;156(5 suppl):1–20.

Back AL, Arnold RM, Baile WF, et al. Approaching difficult communication tasks in oncology. *CA Cancer J Clin*. 2005;55:164–177.

Groves JE. Taking care of the hateful patient. *NEJM*. 1978;298:883–887.

Shaw RJ, DeMaso DR. *Clinical Manual of Pediatric Psychosomatic Medicine: Mental Health Consultation with Physically Ill Children and Adolescents*. Arlington, VA: American Psychiatric Publishing; 2006.

Shemesh E, Yehuda R, Rockmore L, et al. Assessment of depression in medically ill children presenting to pediatric specialty clinics. *JAACAP*. 2005;44(12):1249–1257.

c h a p t e r   1 5

Pulmonary Complications

Reshma Amin and Hartmut Grasemann

Outline

- Life-Threatening Respiratory Emergencies
- Other Pulmonary Complications

Life-Threatening Respiratory Emergencies

- Differential diagnosis:
  - Severe upper airway obstruction (superior vena cava syndrome and superior mediastinal syndrome).
  - Acute respiratory distress syndrome (ARDS)/pneumonia.
  - Pulmonary hemorrhage.
  - Pulmonary edema.

- ○ Pulmonary embolism.
- ○ Status asthmaticus.
- ○ Tension pneumothorax.
- ○ Methemoglobinemia.
- Management:
  - ○ Resuscitation, as indicated.
  - ○ Careful examination with attention to level of consciousness (LOC), vitals, and oxygen saturation.
  - ○ Apply oxygen if respiratory distress.
  - ○ Continuous oxygen saturation monitoring.
  - ○ Assess if any urgent intervention needed.
  - ○ Chest x-ray (CXR).
  - ○ Capillary blood gases, CBC, INR and PTT, electrolytes (Na, K, ionized Ca, Mg), glucose and serum methemoglobin level (if indicated by history → see below).
  - ○ IV access.
  - ○ ECG and echocardiogram.
  - ○ Further management as directed by findings (see below for specific management for each condition).
- Red flags:
  - ○ Any change in level of consciousness (e.g., confusion, agitation).
  - ○ Inability to speak because of dyspnea.
  - ○ Stridor at rest.
  - ○ Bradycardia.
  - ○ Cyanosis.
  - ○ Diaphoresis.
  - ○ Silent chest.
  - ○ Capillary or arterial $Po_2 < 60$ mmHg in room air.
  - ○ $Pco_2 > 50$ mmHg and pH < 7.4.
  - ○ If respiratory distress and any of above → consult pediatric intensive care unit (PICU) and/or activate code blue.

Superior Vena Cava Syndrome and Superior Mediastinal Syndrome

- **Etiology:** Intrathoracic mediastinal tumor, extrathoracic neck tumor, central venous line occlusion/venous thrombosis, chest infection (e.g., Aspergillus).
- **Clinical presentation:** Dyspnea, cough, hoarseness, chest pain, headache, distorted vision, facial swelling, wheeze, stridor, cyanosis or plethora of face, neck and upper extremities.
- **CXR:**
  - Mediastinal mass.
  - Widened mediastinum.
  - Tracheal compression or deviation.
  - May have pericardial and/or pleural effusion.
- **Management:**
  - *Do not lie flat* (keep head of bed at 45°).
  - *Do not sedate.*

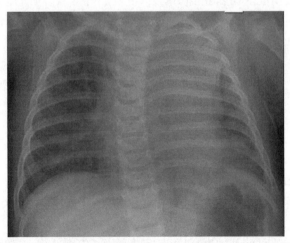

Figure 15-1 Frontal chest radiograph of an Anterior Mediastinal Mass with significant tracheal compression and rightward deviation.
http://www.radpod.org/wp-content/CXRAY28OCT.JPG.

○ Inform anesthesia and PICU about potential critical airway.

○ IV access in lower limbs only.

○ If hemodynamic compromise, consult cardiology for urgent echocardiogram.

○ If critical airway, impending respiratory arrest → consider treatment with prednisone 40 mg/m^2/day:

■ Monitor and treat for tumor lysis syndrome (see Nephrology chapter).

○ Once stable, CT chest and investigate for underlying cause.

Pneumonia/ARDS

- **Etiology:** Infection with bacteria, viruses, mycobacteria (TB and atypical mycobacteria), fungus (Aspergillus, Mucor, Rhizopus), *Pneumocystis jirovecii* (PJP, previously called *Pneumocystis carinii* or PCP).

- **Clinical presentation:** Fever, dyspnea, cough, chest pain, sputum production, hypoxemia, crackles, decreased air entry, asymptomatic.

- **CXR:**
  ○ Focal consolidation or diffuse alveolar disease.
  ○ Pulmonary nodules.
  ○ Cavitating lesions.
  ○ Pleural effusion.
  ○ Hilar adenopathy.

- **Investigations:**
  ○ CBC and differential (high risk if absolute neutrophil count < 0.5/mm^3).
  ○ Capillary blood gases (if severe respiratory distress).

- Nasopharyngeal swab for viruses and pertussis.
- Sputum: Gram stain and culture, fungal stain and culture, silver stain and calcofluor white stain (for PJP), acid-fast bacilli stain and mycobacteria culture, routine respiratory viruses, human herpes viruses, mycoplasma PCR.
- Induced sputum (if not spontaneously productive) → call respiratory therapy for assistance.
- Serologic markers such as LDH and β-D-glucan may be useful for PJP diagnosis.
- Bronchoscopy and bronchoalveolar lavage needs respiratory medicine consult.
- **Further investigations:**
  - Consider TB skin test.
  - Chest ultrasound to quantify amount and type of pleural effusion (e.g., loculated or nonloculated).
  - CT chest if concerned about fungus or interstitial changes on CXR.
  - Consider echocardiogram to look for vegetations (septic emboli), pulmonary pressures (pulmonary hypertension), and ejection fraction (LV failure).
- **Management:**
  - ABCs and oxygen.
  - Broad-spectrum IV antibiotics; consider antifungal coverage if prolonged neutropenia or suggestive imaging; antivirals if viral pathogen identified; high-dose SMX-TMP (cotrimoxazole) IV for empiric treatment or proven PJP.
  - Confirm if patient receiving or adherent to PJP prophylaxis.
  - *Urgent respiratory medicine consult for bronchoscopy.*

○ Chest tube for large pleural effusion, empyema, mediastinal shift, and respiratory distress.

○ Close cardiorespiratory monitoring with timely PICU consult and transfer.

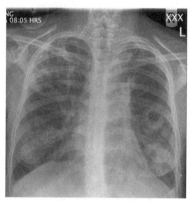

Figure 15-2a Frontal chest radiograph demonstrating multiple cavitary lesions secondary to Invasive Aspergillosis.
Courtesy of Diagnostic Imaging, The Hospital for Sick Children, Toronto.

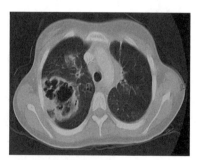

Figure 15-2b Axial Computed Tomographic image of the same patient as Figure 15-2a demonstrating multiple cavitary lesions secondary to Invasive Aspergillosis.
Courtesy of Diagnostic Imaging, The Hospital for Sick Children, Toronto.

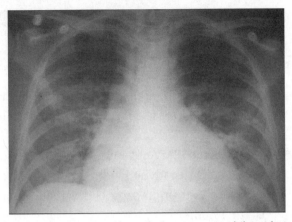

Figure 15-3   Frontal chest radiograph demonstrating bilateral perihilar opacities in a patient with PJP pneumonia.
Published with permission from LearningRadiology.com. (http://www .learningradiology.com/caseofweek/caseoftheweekpix/cow43.jpg)

Pulmonary Hemorrhage

- **Etiology:** Infection (fungal, viral, bacterial, or TB), coagulopathy, septic emboli, pulmonary hypertension, pulmonary embolism, interstitial lung disease, drug toxicity, diffuse alveolar hemorrhage postbone marrow transplant (BMT).
- **Clinical presentation:** Hemoptysis (massive if > 250 ml/24 h), dyspnea, fatigue, crackles, or normal respiratory exam.
- **Management:**
  - Rule out bleeding from GI tract and epistaxis.
  - ABCs and ensure IV access × 2.
  - Continuous oxygen saturation and cardiac monitoring.
  - Stop all anticoagulant medications (e.g., heparin, NSAIDS).

- ○ Stat CBC with cross-match, coagulation profile, and capillary blood gases.
- ○ If hypotensive or massive hemoptysis: Fluid resuscitation with normal saline 20 cc/kg boluses (if no improvement after three boluses, may require PICU admission for inotropic support but continue to fluid bolus until transferred).
- ○ Cross-matched, CMV-negative, irradiated blood transfusion (use O-negative blood if emergent). Dose: 15 cc/kg (rate determined by clinical situation: from push to 4 hours).
- ○ IV vitamin K (10 mg × 1) if coagulapathic; may be given SC to reduce risk of anaphylaxis.
- ○ Stat CXR: Patchy or diffuse alveolar infiltrates.
- ○ Contact PICU for patient transfer.
- ○ Contact respiratory medicine service for diagnostic bronchoscopy and management.

Note: Think of pulmonary hemorrhage in a patient with anemia out of proportion to oncologic disease, high reticulocyte count, and persistent pulmonary infiltrates (high risk if pulmonary hypertension).

Pulmonary Edema

- • **Etiology:**
  - ○ Increased permeability (acute respiratory distress syndrome, sepsis, chemotherapy agents [refer to Table 15-3]).
  - ○ Increased hydrostatic pressure (iatrogenic volume overload, venous hypertension, congestive heart failure secondary to drug toxicity or infection).
  - ○ Impaired lymphatic drainage (malignancy, SVC syndrome).

○ Decreased oncotic pressure (cirrhosis, nephrotic syndrome).

○ Decreased pleural space pressure (reexpansion pulmonary edema).

○ Other (neurogenic pulmonary edema, PE).

- **Clinical presentation:** Dyspnea, cough, fatigue, malaise, nausea, tachypnea, crackles, S3 or S4, hepatomegaly, peripheral edema.

- **Investigations:**

  ○ CXR: Peribronchial cuffing, hyperinflation (early), perihilar opacities, cardiomegaly, Kerley B lines, pleural effusions.

  ○ Echocardiogram to assess ejection fraction.

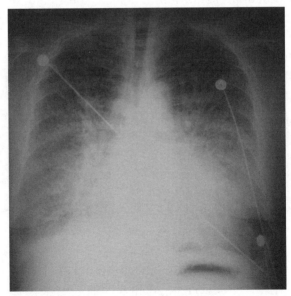

Figure 15-4 Frontal chest radiograph of pulmonary edema demonstrating cardiomegaly, bilateral opacification, obscuring of the right costophrenic angle.

http://www.rad.msu.edu/Education/pages/ Stu_Resources/Common/pages/Aben/ IM_tutor/pages/steps/step6.htm.

- **Management:**
  - Elevate head of bed.
  - Apply oxygen to keep peripheral oxygen saturation > 92%.
  - Diuretics (Lasix 1 mg/kg IV challenge × 1 and assess effect).
  - Limit sodium and fluid intake.

Pulmonary Embolism

- **Etiology:** Hypercoagulability secondary to malignancy, central venous line thromboembolism, cardiac valve vegetation, extremity deep venous thrombosis, prolonged immobility (postsurgery).
- **Clinical presentation:** Dyspnea, chest pain, hemoptysis, hypoxemia, leg swelling, back or shoulder pain, syncope, DIC or asymptomatic.
- **Investigations:**
  - Capillary blood gases (may be normal).
  - CXR:
    - Usually abnormal but with nonspecific findings.
    - Westermark's sign: Oligemia distal to the occluded vessel.
    - Hampton's hump: Focal consolidation in the costophrenic angle.
    - Elevation of the hemi diaphragm.
    - Atelectasis.
    - Consolidation.
  - EKG (right heart strain, tall peaked P-waves in lead II, right axis deviation, right bundle branch block, or S1-Q3-T3 pattern).
  - High-resolution spiral CT chest (filling defect in one of the pulmonary arteries) or ventilation-perfusion (V/Q) nuclear medicine scan (to look for V/Q mismatch).

- D-dimers (not sensitive or specific enough to rule PE in or out).
- Leg Dopplers.
- Ultrasound of central line.
- Pulmonary angiogram is the gold standard.
- **Management:**
  - ABCs and apply oxygen.
  - Assess bleeding risk of patient and consult hematology or thrombosis service for potential anticoagulation.

Airways Hyperreactivity/Status Asthmaticus

- **Etiology:**
  - Personal or family history of asthma and atopy.
  - Exacerbation triggered by chemotherapy (see Table 15-3).
  - Exacerbation triggered by viral infection, allergy (drugs, allergens such as grass pollen, ragweed, dust mites, cats) or exposure to irritants.
- **Clinical presentation:** Dyspnea at rest or with activity, inability to speak, chest pain, change in level of consciousness, prolonged expiratory phase, wheeze, decreased air entry, silent chest.
- **Investigations:**
  - Peripheral oxygen saturation.
  - Capillary blood gases.
  - CXR: Hyperinflation, atelectasis, peribronchial thickening.
- **Management:**
  - Apply oxygen: Keep peripheral oxygen saturation > 92%.
  - Continuous cardiorespiratory monitoring.
  - If significant respiratory distress, NPO and attain IV access.

- Ventolin (0.03 ml/kg plus 3 ml normal saline nebulized). Start by giving 3 back-to-back masks and then titrate frequency according to need (alternatively salbutamol 400 ug by MDI with spacer [aerochamber]).
- IV methylprednisolone (1 mg/kg/dose q 6 h) or PO prednisone (1–2 mg/kg PO) depending on severity.
- Capillary blood gases (if signs of respiratory acidosis call PICU).
- If no improvement after ventolin masks and steroids, will need PICU transfer for further management.
- Follow serum potassium for ventolin-induced hypokalemia.

Tension Pneumothorax

- **Etiology:** Complication of central venous line insertion, pneumothorax from pulmonary metastasis and parenchymal erosion, radiation, initial presentation of pleuropulmonary blastoma, Langerhan's cell histiocytosis, or sarcoma.
- **Clinical presentation:** Respiratory distress or arrest, dyspnea, chest pain, deviated trachea, decreased or absent air entry, hypotension.
- **Diagnosis:**
  - Mediastinal shift away from affected side.
  - Absence of lung markings on affected side (hyperlucency).
  - Ipsilateral lung edge seen parallel to chest wall.
- **Management:**
  - Management of ABCs and resuscitation as indicated.
  - *Urgent* needle aspiration of affected side.
  - Use 14–16 gauge angiocatheter attached to 3-way stopcock and syringe.

- ○ Locate puncture site (2nd intercostal space midclavicular line superior to the rib).
- ○ Clean site with betadine or alcohol.
- ○ Insert needle and listen for gush of air.
- ○ Remove needle.
- ○ Secure syringe in position.
- ○ Call PICU or general surgery for chest tube insertion.
- ○ Chest tube connected to Pleurovac system and –15 to –20 cmH$_2$O wall suction.
- ○ If cessation of air leak for 24 hours (cessation of bubbling in the Pleurovac system with respiration) take off suction.
- ○ Repeat CXR 6 h later → no reaccumulation → pull tube; if reaccumulates → back on suction.
- ○ Chest tube *does not* have to be clamped before removal with the Pleurovac system.

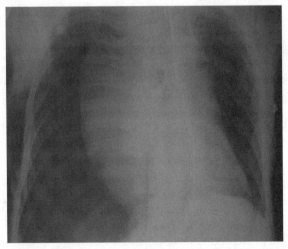

Figure 15-5 Frontal chest radiograph of a tension pneumothorax with complete collapse of the right lung with mediastinal shift to the left.
http://www.aic.cuhk.edu.hk/web8/Hi%20res/ 0229%
20Tension%20pneumothorax.jpg.

Methemoglobinemia

- **Definition:** Iron in hemoglobin is oxidized to the Fe^{+3} state and cannot bind oxygen.
- **Etiology:** Dapsone, cotrimoxazole, antimalarials, rasburicase, nitric oxide, aniline dyes, lidocaine, prilocaine, glucose-6-phosphate dehydrogenase deficiency (G6PD), silver nitrate, and a rare congenital form.
- **Clinical presentation:** Cyanosis, dyspnea, lethargy, headache, dizziness, deterioration of mental functioning, or stupor.
- **Investigations:**
  - Oximetry does not correspond to degree of cyanosis.
  - Blood gas will show a normal Po_2.
  - Serum methemoglobin level ($> 1\%$ is abnormal).
  - Quick bedside test: Bubble 100% oxygen in a tube that contains the patient's blood: If the blood remains dark → methemoglobinemia.
- **Management:**
  - In asymptomatic patients with low levels of methemoglobin → follow serum levels (discontinue offending exposure).
  - If symptomatic and/or methemoglobin levels are more than 30%: Administer methylene blue IV at 1–2 mg/kg (up to 50 mg/dose in adults, adolescents, and older children) as a 1% solution over 5 minutes; repeat in 1 hour, if necessary.
  - Note: Methylene blue is an oxidant at levels of more than 7 mg/kg and may cause methemoglobinemia in susceptible patients; thus, care must be taken in administration of this drug.
  - *Methylene blue is contraindicated in patients with G6PD deficiency because it can lead to severe hemolysis.*

Other Pulmonary Complications

Pleural Effusion

- **Etiology:**
  - Increased permeability (pneumonia or sepsis).
  - Increased hydrostatic pressure (volume overload, venous hypertension, congestive heart failure).
  - Impaired lymphatic drainage (malignancy, SVC syndrome).
  - Decreased oncotic pressure (cirrhosis, nephrotic syndrome).
  - Decreased pleural space pressure (reexpansion pulmonary edema).
- **Symptoms:** Asymptomatic, dyspnea, orthopnea, chest pain, pleuritic pain.
- **Signs:** Pleural rub (will decrease as effusion increases), decreased chest excursion, dullness to percussion, decreased fremitus, decreased breath sounds.
- **CXR:**
  - Partial or complete opacification of affected side and blunting of costophrenic angle.
  - May see meniscus of fluid.
  - Mediastinal shift to contralateral side.
  - Supine films *not* sensitive at detecting pleural effusions → upright or lateral decubitus preferred.
- **Management:**
  - IV antibiotics.
  - Chest ultrasound: Distinguish pleural thickening from nonloculated and loculated effusion.
  - Early thoracocentesis: R/O malignancy and identify micro-organism.
  - Investigations:
    - Pleural fluid: Cell count, differential, glucose, protein, LDH, triglycerides, cytology, gram stain and

culture, fungal stain and culture, PJP calcofluor white stain.

- Serum at same time for CBC, diff., glucose, protein, LDH.
- Differentiate between transudate and exudate (see Table 15-1).

○ Insertion of chest tube when indicated (see Table 15-2).

○ Chest tube to suction (-15 to -20 cmH_2O).

○ Ensure suction adequate: Check that indicator visible in window of Pleurovac system (see Figure 15-6b).

○ Column of water should vary with respiration.

○ There should be no bubbling (bubbling suggests air leak).

○ If Pleurovac system full from drainage, clamp chest tube before disconnecting and connecting new Pleurovac, and then unclamp.

○ If drainage < 30 ml per day and constitutional symptoms resolved, then remove tube.

○ Failure of above → surgical consultation for video-assisted thoracoscopic surgery (VATS).

Table 15-1 Pleural fluid criteria to differentiate exudate and transudate.

Effusion Type	Pleural Liquid Concentration			Pleural/Serum Concentration Ratio	
	pH	Protein	LDH	Protein	LDH
Transudate	> 7.45	< 3g/dl	< 2/3 serum	< 0.5	< 0.6
Exudate	≤ 7.45	≥ 3g/dl	> 2/3 serum	≥ 0.5	≥ 0.6

Source: Adapted with permission from Chernick V, Boat TF, Wilmott RW, Bush A. *Kendig's Disorders of the Respiratory Tract in Children.* 3rd ed. Philadelphia, PA: Elsevier Inc; 2006.

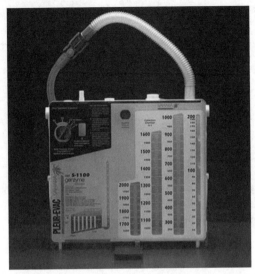

Figure 15-6a   Chest tube set up used at the Hospital for Sick Children. The blue water level in the bottom left of the PLEUR-EVAC® should not bubble, as this would indicate an air leak.
http://www.teleflexmedical.com

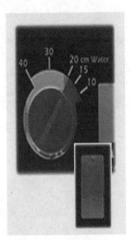

Figure 15-6b   Close up of suction dial and indicator window with adequate suction.
http://www.teleflexmedical.com/ucd/images/figure16.gif.

Table 15-2 Indications for immediate chest tube insertion.

Indications for immediate chest tube insertion
Large effusion causing mediastinal shift and cardio respiratory symptoms
Frank pus in the pleural fluid
Positive gram stain in the pleural fluid
pH < 7.20

Source: Adapted with permission from Chernick V, Boat TF, Wilmott RW, Bush A. *Kendig's Disorders of the Respiratory Tract in Children.* 3rd ed. Philadelphia, PA: Elsevier Inc.; 2006.

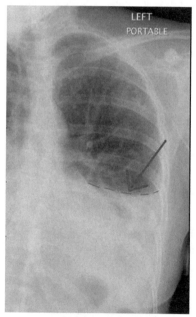

Figure 15-7 Frontal chest radiograph demonstrating a left sided pleural effusion with visual meniscus of fluid (arrow).

http://sprojects.mmi.mcgill.ca/pneumonia/xrays/pleural%20eff%20ans_files/image004.jpg.

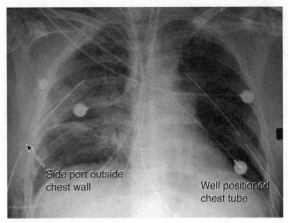

Figure 15-8 Frontal chest radiograph demonstrating a poorly positioned chest tube in the right lung and a well positioned chest tube in the left lung.

Printed with permission from the University of Iowa's virtual hospital.

(http://www.icufaqs.org/ChestTubes.doc)

- **Trouble shooting:** If chest tube drainage stops but large residual effusion:
  - Check tubing: Make sure it is not kinked.
  - Repeat CXR: Ensure tube is in correct position (see Figure 15-8).
  - Try to flush chest tube with 10 ml normal saline.
  - Administer tissue plasminogen activated (t-Pa) for clotted chest tubes.

Bronchiolitis Obliterans

- **Definition:**
  - Obliteration of the lumen of small bronchi and bronchioles causing chronic airway obstruction.
  - Early diagnosis is essential because this disease is irreversible.
  - Early intervention may help prevent progression.

- **Etiology:** Infection (adenovirus, TB, mycoplasma), organ transplantation (following lung transplantation or any organ (e.g., solid and HSCT), drugs (e.g., penicillamine), inflammatory (Stevens-Johnson syndrome, collagen vascular diseases), toxic inhalations.
- **Presentation:** Dyspnea, increased oxygen requirements, may have end expiratory wheeze heard only with forced expiration, exercise intolerance, declining pulmonary function (FEV_1 and FEF_{25-75}).
- **Investigations:**
  ○ Rule out active infection (see pneumonia section).
  ○ CXR.
  ○ High-resolution CT chest with inspiratory and expiratory views.
  ○ Pulmonary function tests (PFTs).
- **Imaging:**
  ○ Hyperinflation, gas trapping.
  ○ Peribronchial thickening or patchy bronchopneumonia.
  ○ Nodular or reticulonodular pattern.
  ○ Mosaic perfusion and air trapping on high-resolution CT chest.
- **Treatment:**
  ○ Pulse methylprednisone (20 mg/kg/day IV × 3 days every month for 6 months) as per discussion with respiratory medicine.
  ○ Regular monitoring of pulmonary function testing (attention to FEV_1 and FEF_{25-75}).
  ○ Azithromycin (consider) for maintenance.

Note: The first sign of bronchiolitis obliterans is usually a drop in the FEF_{25-75}, which is a marker of small airways disease.

Pulmonary Hypertension (PHTN)

- **Etiology:**
  - Pulmonary arterial hypertension (myeloproliferative diseases, drugs).
  - Pulmonary venous hypertension (left-sided atrial, ventricular, or valvular issues).
  - Pulmonary hypertension with hypoxemia (sleep-disordered breathing, alveolar disease).
  - Pulmonary hypertension associated with thromboembolic disease.
  - Other (compression of pulmonary vessels by adenopathy or tumor).
- **Clinical presentation:** Tachypnea, tachycardia, poor appetite, failure to thrive, lethargy, diaphoresis, irritability, cyanosis or dyspnea w/exertion or syncope, peripheral edema, hypoxic seizures, loud S2, murmur of tricuspid regurgitation, right ventricular heave, hepatomegaly, ascites, clubbing.
- **Investigations:**
  - CXR.
  - EKG and echocardiogram.
  - PFTS, overnight oximetry, early morning capillary blood gas.
  - Respiratory medicine and pulmonary hypertension team consult.
- **Management:**
  - ABCs.
  - Keep oxygen saturation $> 92\%$.
  - Use diuretics with caution in patients with RV failure (preload will decrease).
  - Treatment of underlying cause.

Pulmonary Toxicity Due to Chemotherapeutic Agents

- Difficult to diagnose because no pathognomonic findings.

Table 15-3   Cytoxic drugs and pulmonary syndromes.

	Clinical Syndrome
Antibiotics	
Bleomycin	IP/PF, H, P.Eff.
Mitomycin	IP/EF, P.Ed, P.Eff
Alkylating agents	
Cyclophosphamide	IP/PF, P.Ed, B, PH
Chlorambucil	IP/PF
Busulfan	IP/PF, P.Eff
Melphalan	IP/PF
Nitrosureas	
Carmustine	PF
Antimetabolites	
Methotrexate	IP/PF, H, P.Ed, P.Eff
Azathioprine	IP/PF
6-Mercaptopurine	IP/PF
Cystosine arabinoside	IP/PF, P.Ed, BOOP
Gemcitabine	P.Ed
L-Asparaginase	H
Other	
Etoposide (VP-16)	H
Hydroxyurea	H
Paclitaxel	H

Note: B, bronchospasm; BOOP, bronchiolitis obliterans and organizing pneumonia; H, hypersensitivity pneumonitis; IP/PF, interstitial pneumonitis and pulmonary fibrosis; P.Ed., noncardiogenic pulmonary edema; P.Eff., pleural effusion; PF, pulmonary fibrosis; PH, pulmonary hemorrhage.
Source: Adapted with permission from Chernick V, Boat TF, Wilmott RW, Bush A. *Kendig's Disorders of the Respiratory Tract in Children.* 3rd ed. Philadelphia, PA: Elsevier Inc; 2006.

Methotrexate Pulmonary Toxicity

- **Clinical presentation:** Acute pleuritis with fever, malaise, headache, dyspnea, dry cough, tachypnea, crackles, cyanosis, and occasionally skin eruptions.
- **Investigations:**
  ○ CXR: Usually bilateral interstitial infiltrates, but sometimes nodular or alveolar pattern, pleural effusions.
  ○ PFTS: May see a restrictive pattern: Decreased total lung capacity (TLC), decreased forced vital capacity (FVC), decreased diffusion capacity of the lung for carbon monoxide (DLCO).
- **Management:**
  ○ If symptomatic: Systemic steroids (1 mg/kg/day) and once response established → wean slowly.
  ○ Reintroduce methotrexate with great caution!

Bleomycin Toxicity

- Toxicity is usually dose related after cumulative dose of 400 to 450 units but can happen after any amount.
- **Clinical presentation:** Usually insidious onset, fever, dry cough, dyspnea, tachypnea, crackles. May present with acute chest pain syndrome.
- **Investigations:**
  ○ CXR: Reticular-nodular infiltrates that can progress to diffuse interstitial or alveolar infiltrates.
  ○ PFTS: Diffusing capacity of the lung for carbon monoxide (DLCO) decreases first and then forced vital capacity (FVC) and then total lung capacity (TLC).
  ○ CT: More sensitive than CXR.
- **Management:**
  ○ Minimize supplemental oxygen to treat hypoxemia of any cause for patients previously treated with

bleomycin (oxygen toxicity synergistic with bleomycin toxicity).

○ Avoid further treatment involving bleomycin.
○ If symptomatic: Systemic steroids (1 mg/kg/day) and once response established → wean slowly.
○ Follow with serial PFTS and chest CT.

Radiation Pneumonitis

- **Etiology:** Direct chest or mantle radiation therapy.
- **Clinical presentation:**
  ○ Usually 1–4 months after the completion of radiation treatment.
  ○ Nonproductive cough, low-grade fever, gradual onset of exercise-induced dyspnea.
  ○ May progress to acute respiratory failure (can be fatal).
  ○ May progress to chronic fibrosis which develops 9–12 months postirradiation.

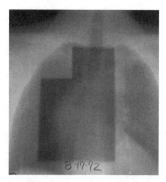

Figure 15-9a Frontal chest radiograph showing location of radiation exposure field.

Published with permission from LearningRadiology.com.

(http://www.learningradiology.com/toc/tocsubsection/tocarchives2003.htm)

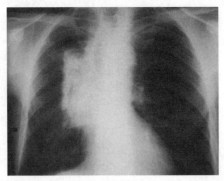

Figure 15-9b Frontal chest radiograph showing evidence of radiation pneumonitis.
Published with permission from LearningRadiology.com.
(http://www.learningradiology.com/toc/tocsubsection/tocarchives2003.htm)

- **Investigations:**
  - ○ CXR: Patchy infiltrates and nonanatomical border corresponding to the edge of the radiation port or infiltrates in contralateral lung, pleural effusion.
- **Management:** Systemic steroids (1 mg/kg OD) for symptomatic patients with slow taper over months.

References

Cheng A, Williams B, Sivarajan VB. *Hospital for Sick Children Handbook*. 10th ed. Toronto, Canada: Elsevier Inc.; 2003.

Chernick V, Boat TF, Wilmott RW, Bush A. *Kendig's Disorders of the Respiratory Tract in Children*. 3rd ed. Philadelphia, PA: Elsevier Inc.; 2006.

Meyer S, Reinhard H, Gottschling S. Pulmonary dysfunction in pediatric oncology patients. *Pediatr Hematol*. 2004;21:175–195.

Stover D, Kaner R. Pulmonary complications in cancer patients. *CA-A Cancer J Clinic*. 1996;46(5):303–320.

Renal Complications

Tony H. Truong, Ronald Grant, and Valerie Langlois

Outline

- Tumor Lysis Syndrome
- Electrolyte Abnormalities
- Hypertension
- Hematuria
- Acute Renal Failure

Tumor Lysis Syndrome

- A group of electrolyte derangements resulting from abrupt and massive breakdown of malignant cells and the release of intracellular contents into the circulation.
- Laboratory tumor lysis syndrome (TLS) is defined as any two or more laboratory changes within 3 days before or 7 days after chemotherapy initiation:
  - Hyperkalemia ≥ 6.0 mmol/l or 25% increase from baseline.

- ○ Hyperuricemia ≥ 475 mmol/l or 25% increase from baseline.
- ○ Hyperphosphatemia ≥ 2.1 mmol/l or 25% increase from baseline.
- ○ Hypocalcemia ≤ 1.75 mmol/l or 25% decrease from baseline.
- ○ Renal insufficiency.
- Rarely does laboratory TLS lead to clinical TLS (renal failure, cardiac arrhythmia, or seizure).

Risk Factors

Patients can be stratified into three risk categories:

- High risk:
  - ○ Children with newly diagnosed/relapsed Burkitt's lymphoma.
  - ○ Children who present with:
    - A white blood cell count (WBC) ≥ 50 × 10^9/l.
    - Serum urate concentrations > 475 μmol/l; or
    - Preexisting renal impairment, prolonged use of ibuprofen, dehydration or septic shock.
    - Serum lactate dehydrogenase (LDH) concentration > 2000 U/l.
    - Evidence of increased tumor burden: mediastinal mass, bulky lymphadenopathy, or hepatosplenomegaly.
  - ○ Children with T-cell ALL, T-cell lymphoblastic lymphoma, or precursor B-cell ALL.
- Low risk: Patients in this category must have all three of the following proposed criteria:
  - ○ Age < 10 years *and*
  - ○ Initial WBC ≤ 20 × 10^9/l *and*
  - ○ No evidence of a mediastinal mass or splenomegaly.

- Intermediate risk: Identifying criteria are yet to be determined, but generally are those who do not belong in either the high-risk or low-risk groups.

Investigations

- CBC with differential.
- Serum creatinine, urea, urate, sodium, potassium, chloride, phosphate, calcium, albumin, total carbon dioxide (TCO_2), LDH concentrations.
- If albumin is low, check serum ionized calcium concentration.
- Check electrolytes and uric acid every 4–6 hours in high-risk patients or every 8–12 hours in low-risk patients initially.
- Measure accurate urine output, urine specific gravity, and urine pH.

Prevention and Management

Tumor lysis syndrome is prevented and managed by hyperhydration, antiurate agents, and correction of electrolyte abnormalities.

Hyperhydration

- Administer IV hydration.
  - Until serum electrolyte values are known, administer 0.9% sodium chloride (normal saline) at 3 l/m^2/day (or 200 ml/kg/day if child weighs ≤ 10 kg). The addition of dextrose may be necessary based on the child's age, blood glucose level, and clinical condition.
  - Monitor the serum sodium (Na^+) concentration (along with tumor lysis laboratory monitoring) to

avoid hyper/hyponatremia, especially in the setting of impaired urine output. If serum $Na^+ = 138–144$ mmol/l, changing the IV solution to 0.45% NaCl (1/2 normal saline) may be considered.

○ Do not give potassium, calcium, or phosphate in hydration fluids, at least initially, unless patient is symptomatic.

○ Hydration should begin 24 to 48 hours prior to administration of antineoplastic therapy.

• Maintain fluid balance:

○ Total fluid intake (TFI) = urine output + insensible losses (400 ml/m^2/day in an afebrile child) + other losses.

• Ensure adequate urine output:

○ Administer furosemide or mannitol to maintain a urine output of at least 2.4 l/m^2/day (at least 160 ml/kg/day in patients $\leq$ 10 kg).

○ The maximum tolerated positive fluid balance in an afebrile patient is 600 ml/m^2/day. Diuretics should be avoided when contraindicated (e.g., in the presence of hypovolemia).

○ Check each void and maintain urine specific gravity less $\leq$ 1.010.

• Assess weight daily.

Urine Alkalinization

• At a low acidic pH, uric acid crystallizes in renal tubules. At a high alkaline pH, xanthine and hypoxanthine may crystallize. As well, calcium phosphate precipitation is more likely at higher urine pH values.

• Alkalinization, although still widely used, has been abandoned by some institutions (including the Hospital for Sick Children, Toronto) due to the potential risks of nephrocalcinosis and metabolic alkalosis, as well as the lack of evidence for its efficacy.

- There is no consensus on the use of alkalinization for intermediate-risk patients; for low-risk patients, and high-risk patients (requiring rasburicase) → alkalinization may not be required.
- Alkalinization may be considered only for patients with metabolic acidosis.

Antiurate Agents

- For patients at high risk of developing TLS, administer urate oxidase or rasburicase:
  - Dose: 0.2 mg/kg/dose IV over 30 minutes q 24 h, as needed.
  - Rasburicase is a recombinant form of urate oxidase that catalyzes the conversion of uric acid into allantoin (readily soluble and excreted in the urine).
  - Unlike allopurinol, rasburicase reduces preexisting uric acid.
  - Rasburicase is contraindicated in patients with G6PD deficiency, as it may cause acute hemolytic anemia. In male patients, send blood immediately for G6PD assay prior to giving rasburicase (do not wait for results prior to giving rasburicase).
  - Send all urate samples *on ice* for 96 hours following urate oxidase administration (samples at room temperature will be lower than actual).
  - The use of rasburicase negates the need for urine alkalinization.
- Other indications for rasburicase:
  - Children who cannot take oral medications for physiological reasons (intractable vomiting, impaired gastrointestinal absorption).

○ Children who present with significant renal impairment (serum creatinine ≥ 1.5 times the upper limit of normal for age).

○ Children with newly diagnosed/relapsed malignancy with significant hyperuricemia (> 475 μmol/l), despite oral allopurinol administration for at least 48 hours.

○ Children who have developed allergic reactions to allopurinol.

○ Note: Antibodies to rasburicase are known to develop. All patients receiving this agent should be monitored for signs and symptoms of an allergic response. Patients who are retreated with rasburicase following a relapse may be at increased risk of developing hypersensitivity reactions.

• For patients who do not receive rasburicase, administer allopurinol:

○ Dose: 200–300 mg/m^2/day PO div BID–QID or 12 mg/kg/day PO div BID–QID

○ Allopurinol inhibits xanthine oxidase and prevents the metabolism of xanthine and hypoxanthine to uric acid.

○ Allopurinol should be continued for at least 72 hours after the initiation of antineoplastic therapy and then discontinued only when serum urate concentrations are within normal limits and stable.

Electrolyte Abnormalities

Basics of Fluid and Electrolyte Administration

• Assess the patient's fluid status and administer fluids accordingly.

- Examine for clinical signs of dehydration.
- Oncology patients are at risk for increased renal injury given exposure to multiple chemotherapeutic agents, antibiotics, and antifungals.
- Calculate maintenance IV fluids and replace ongoing nonrenal fluid losses.
- If patient is receiving chemotherapy, consult the protocol to ensure proper type and rate of IV fluids.
- Record urine output and specific gravity when indicated.
- Situations that require increased hydration:
  o Tumor lysis prevention.
  o Certain chemotherapy agents: Methotrexate, cyclophosphamide, ifosfamide, cisplatin, others.
  o Dehydration.
  o Fever.

Hyponatremia

Etiology

- Hypovolemic: Extracellular fluid (ECF) volume contraction:
  o Renal:
    - Mineralocorticoid deficiency.
    - Diuretics.
    - Polyuric acute renal failure.
    - Salt-wasting renal disease.
  o Gastrointestinal: Diarrhea.
  o Third space: Septic shock, burns, trauma.
- Euvolemic: normal ECF volume:
  o Glucocorticoid deficiency.
  o Hypothyroidism.
  o Hypotonic IV fluids.

- Normal or hypervolemic: ECF volume expansion:
  - Syndrome of inappropriate ADH secretion (SIADH).
  - Acute renal failure.
  - Nephrotic syndrome.
  - Hepatic cirrhosis.
  - Congestive heart failure.
  - Compulsive drinking.
- *Consider pseudohyponatremia* causes: Hyperglycemia, mannitol, hyperproteinemia, hyperlipidemia.

Clinical Manifestations of Acute Hyponatremia

- Asymptomatic, lethargy, headache, nausea, vomiting, irritability, obtundation, seizures, apnea, coma.

Investigations

- Serum: Electrolytes, creatinine, urea, osmolarity.
- Urine: Electrolytes, creatinine, and osmolarity.
- Monitor intake and output.

Management

- Goal is to normalize the Na^+ and manage the underlying cause.
- In general:
  - Hypovolemia: Give Na^+.
  - Euvolemia or hypervolemia: Restrict free water.
  - Monitor the serum Na^+ frequently and adjust fluid accordingly.
  - In emergency situations such as seizures, give NaCl 3% (2–3 ml/kg) rapidly.
  - In nonacute settings, calculate Na deficit = (Na desired – Na actual) $\times$ 0.6 $\times$ Wt (kg) = mmol Na to give over 24–48 h (rate of increase in sodium should be about 10–12 mmol/day) → this amount of sodium should be given in addition to maintenance requirements.

Hypernatremia

Etiology

- Hypovolemic hypernatremia:
  - GI losses: Vomiting, diarrhea.
  - Renal losses: Excess free water loss, diuretics, osmotic diuresis (hyperglycemia, mannitol).
  - Increased insensible loss.
  - Poor water intake.
- Euvolemia:
  - Nephrogenic diabetes insipidus, central diabetes insipidus.
- Hypervolemic hypernatremia:
  - Hypertonic IV fluid administration.
  - High Na intake.
  - Hyperaldosteronism.

Clinical Manifestations

- Thirst, irritability, lethargy, weakness, seizures, coma.

Investigations

- Serum electrolytes, creatinine, urea, osmolarity.
- Urine: Electrolytes, creatinine, and osmolarity.
- Monitor intake and output.

Management

- Differentiate patients with water deficit versus those with salt intoxication.
- Administer fluid to lower the serum Na by no more than 10–12 mmol/l/day (for patients with free-water deficit).
- Rapid correction of hypernatremia can cause potentially fatal cerebral edema:
  - Close monitoring of electrolytes and CNS status.

Hypokalemia

Etiology

- Poor intake of K^+:
  - Poor diet and nutrition.
  - GI malabsorption.
- Increased K+ loss:
  - Increased urinary losses: Amphotericin, aminoglycosides, penicillin, diuretics, hyperaldosteronism.
  - Increased gastrointestinal losses: Vomiting, diarrhea.
- Shift of K+ to the intracellular compartment:
  - Bicarbonate infusion, insulin, β_2 agonist.

Clinical Manifestations

- Cardiac: ↓ST segments, ↓T-waves, U-waves, ↑QT intervals, ventricular fibrillation (VF), other arrhythmias.
- Muscle: Weakness, cramp, myalgia, restless leg syndrome, rhabdomyolysis, respiratory failure.

Investigations

- Laboratory: Serum Na^+, K^+, chloride, Mg^+, creatinine, osmolality, blood gases; urine Na^+, K^+, chloride, creatinine, osmolality, and pH.
- Monitor intake and output.
- ECG.

Management

- Treat underlying cause.
- Replace K^+ in maintenance IV fluids to meet daily requirements.
- Administer K^+ via intermittent, slow bolus infusions:
  - Dose: 0.2–0.5 mmol/kg/h.
  - Repeat the K^+ after each bolus to ensure a response.

- Warning: Do not exceed maximum rates of IV K^+ administration (0.5 mmol/kg/h via CVL). ECG monitoring is required for administering rates greater than or equal to 0.2 mmol/kg/h.

Hyperkalemia

Etiology

- Falsely elevated potassium:
  - Sampling error: Inadequate blood withdrawn from central venous line.
  - Hemolysed sample.
  - Extreme thrombocytosis, leukocytosis.
- Increased intake:
  - Excessive oral or IV K+ given.
  - Blood transfusion.
- Decreased renal excretion:
  - Obstructive uropathy.
  - Renal failure.
  - Hypoaldosteronism.
  - Adrenal insufficiency.
- Shift from intracellular to extracellular:
  - Tumor lysis syndrome.
  - Rhabdomyolysis.

Clinical Manifestations

- Cardiac: Tall and peaked T-waves, decreased amplitude of P-waves, QRS widening, VT, VF, any arrhythmia on ECG.
- ECG changes generally correlate with potassium levels, but life-threatening arrhythmias may occur with any degree of hyperkalemia.

Investigations

- Serum Na^+, K^+, chloride, Mg^+, creatinine, osmolality, blood gases; urine Na^+, K^+, chloride, creatinine, osmolality and pH; may add CPK and CBC/blood smear.
- Calculate the trans-tubular K^+ gradient (TTKG):
  ○ TTKG = (urine K^+ / plasma K^+) / (Urine Osm/Plasma Osm).
  ○ A TTKG < 6 during hyperkalemia suggests hypoaldosteronism.
- Monitor intake and output of fluids.
- ECG.

Management

- Resuscitate as indicated.
- Cardiac monitoring.
- Stop any K^+ infusion or supplementation.
- Repeat K+ level immediately.
- Stabilize myocardium: Calcium gluconate 10% solution (0.5 ml/kg IV over 5–10 minutes).
- Shift K+ intracellular:
  ○ Salbutamol: 0.03 ml/kg nebulized $\times$ 3 times consecutively.
  ○ $NaHCO_3$: 1–2 mmol/kg IV over 30 minutes.
  ○ dextrose with insulin bolus: 0.5–1 g/kg glucose and insulin 0.1–0.2 units/kg; continuous infusion: dextrose 10% 5 ml/kg/hr and insulin 0.1 unit/kg/h.
- Promote K+ clearance: Diuretics or potassium-binding resin: kayexelate 1 gm/kg PO/PR.
- If all else fails: dialysis.

Hypophosphatemia

Etiology

- Increased urinary phosphate loss.

- Decreased gastrointestinal phosphate absorption.
- Phosphate shifts from extracellular to intracellular compartment.

Clinical Manifestations

- Asymptomatic.
- Chronic severe hypophosphatemia (phosphate < 0.35 mmol/l): muscle weakness and myalgia.

Investigations

- Serum Na^+, K^+, Cl^-, creatinine, phosphate, Ca^{2+}, pH, HCO_3^-, PTH, vitamin D.
- Urine phosphate, Ca^{2+}, creatinine.

Management

- Replace phosphate by oral supplementation preferable; some patients unable to tolerate oral meds will require IV phosphate.
- Oral therapy: 1–2 mmol/kg/day by mouth divided two to four times daily.
- IV therapy: 1–2 mmol phosphate/kg/day IV in divided doses.

Hyperphosphatemia

Etiology

- Decreased urinary phosphate loss: Renal failure.
- Increased gastrointestinal phosphate absorption.
- Phosphate shifts from intracellular to extracellular compartment: Tumor lysis syndrome.
- Drugs: Amphotericin-B.

Clinical Manifestations

- Asymptomatic.

- Often associated with hypocalcemia.
- Phosphate may precipitate with calcium and cause metastatic calcifications or renal failure.

Investigations

- Serum Na^+, K^+, Cl^-, creatinine, phosphate, Ca^{2+}, blood gases, PTH, vitamin D.
- CBC/differential/smear, CPK.
- Urine phosphate, Ca^{2+}, creatinine, urine dipstick (for tumor lysis, hemoglobinuria, or myoglobinuria).

Management

- Treat underlying cause.
- Hold any IV phosphate.
- Reduce GI absorption:
  ○ Decrease dietary phosphate intake.
  ○ Phosphate binders: Sevelamer hydrochloride.
- Increase phosphate urinary excretion with volume expansion.
- Dialysis in severe situations.

Hypomagnesemia

Etiology

- Increased Mg^{2+} losses:
  ○ Chemotherapy: Cisplatin, cyclosporine.
  ○ Other medications: Amphotericin, aminoglycosides, foscarnet, ethanol, loop and thiazides diuretics.
- Decreased Mg^{2+} absorption or intake.

Clinical Manifestations

- Usually asymptomatic.

- Cardiac ECG: Prolonged QT, Torsade de pointes, arrhythmia.
- Often seen in combination with hypokalemia and/or hypocalcemia.

Investigations
- Laboratory: Plasma Mg^{2+}, K^+, Ca^{2+}, creatinine, albumin
- Urine Mg^{2+}, Ca^{2+}, creatinine.
- Monitor intake and output.

Management
- Oral Mg^{2+} supplements 20–40 mg elemental magnesium/kg/day in divided doses (to minimize diarrhea).
- Parenteral treatment: 5–10 mg elemental magnesium/kg/dose.
- Consider adding Mg in IV fluids or in TPN.

Hypertension

- Definition: A systolic or diastolic blood pressure persistently above the 95th percentile for gender, age, and height.

Etiology
- Renal: Primary renal parenchymal disease, renal artery stenosis, compression from an external mass:
  - Wilms' tumor, neuroblastoma, abdominal lymphomas.
- Ectopic renin production: Wilms' tumor, neuroblatoma.
- Renal vein thrombosis.
- Increased ICP results in Cushing triad: Hypertension, bradycardia, and respiratory depression.

- Fluid overload.
- Pain, anxiety.
- Medications: Steroids, cyclosporine A, β_2 agonists.

Clinical Presentation

- Can be aymptomatic.
- Headache, irritability, lethargy, confusion, and if severe, seizures, and coma.
- Complications: Intracranial hemorrhage.

Investigation

- Serum sodium, potassium, chloride, urea, creatinine, calcium.
- Urine analysis.
- 4-limb blood pressure: Rule out (R/O) coarctation of the aorta.
- ECG and CXR: Look for signs of LVH or cardiomegaly.
- Abdominal US with Doppler.
- Urine and plasma catecholamines.
- CT scan of head (if increased ICP suspected), or ultrasound/CT abdomen (to rule out abdominal mass).

Treatment

- Treat the underlying cause.
- Short-acting PRN medications:
  ○ Hydralazine 0.15–0.8 mg/kg/dose IV q 4–6 h.
  ○ Nifedipine SL 0.25–0.5 mg/kg/dose PO q 4 h PRN, bite and swallow.
- If patient is fluid overloaded, give furosemide (1.0 mg/kg/dose); decrease IV fluids if applicable.
- For increased ICP: Dexamethasone or mannitol.

- For persistent/chronic hypertension: Consult pediatric nephrology; consider treatment with calcium-channel blocking agents (e.g., amlodipine), ACE-inhibitors (e.g., enalapril or captopril) or β-blockers.
- For hypertensive emergency: Transfer to PICU; use continuous infusion of a β-blocker or a vasodilator.

Complications

- Congestive heart failure.
- Stroke, intracranial hemorrhage.
- Encephalopathy: PRES syndrome (see Chapter 11).

Hematuria

Etiology

- Drugs:
  - Hemorrhagic cystitis:
    - Cyclophosphamide or ifosfamide (may occur hours to months after administration).
    - Acrolein, the principal metabolite of these drugs, is damaging to uroepithelial cells when excreted in the urine.
- Infections:
  - Bacteria.
  - Adenovirus.
  - CMV.
  - Polyomavirus BK.
- Hypercalciuria and renal stones:
  - Secondary to steroids.
- Renal-invading tumor: Wilms tumor, renal cell carcinoma.
- Renal vein thrombosis.

- Coagulation abnormality (DIC); severe thrombocytopenia.
- Sickle cell nephropathy.
- Acute glomerulonephritis.
- Bladder malignancy: Rhabdomyosarcoma.

Clinical Presentation

- Pink to red to dark brown (cola-colored) urine.
- Blood clots.
- Dysuria, urgency, frequency.

Investigations

- Urine: Microscopy, cultures, viruses.
- Serum electrolytes, calcium, phosphate, total CO_2, creatinine, urea.
- CBC, blood smear.
- Doppler US bladder: May demonstrate edematous bladder and to examine blood flow.
- If renal stones are suspected, check urine calcium, oxalate, citrate, urate, and creatinine.

Management

The following section applies to the management of hemorrhagic cystitis:

- Best prevented with hydration pre- and post-cyclophosphamide.
- Use of MESNA: Sodium 2-mercaptoethane sulfonate; a uroprotective agent that binds acrolein.

- Acute management:
  - Increase hydration.
  - Correction of thrombocytopenia and coagulopathies.
  - Increase diuresis: use of furosemide.
  - Bladder irrigation with normal saline: placement of Foley catheter.
- Patients who continue to bleed may need urology consultation for management:
  - Cystoscopy to identify bleeding site.
  - Electrocoagulation.
  - Instillation of agents: Formalin (used in past; contraindicated in patients with urinary reflux) and now prostaglandin E_2 (PGE2).

For other etiologies of hematuria, identify and treat the underlying cause.

Acute Renal Failure

Etiology

- Prerenal:
  - True hypovolemia:
    - GI losses (infectious diarrhea, chemotherapy-induced emesis).
    - Hemorrhage.
    - Renal losses (diabetes mellitus or insipidus, diuretics).
    - Poor intake.
  - Decreased effective circulating volume:
    - Sepsis: Most common.
    - Third space losses (abdominal surgery, ascites, pancreatitis).
    - Heart failure.

- Intrinsic renal failure:
  - Preexisting diseases of the kidney:
    - Polycystic kidney disease.
    - Any structural abnormality (horseshoe kidney, solitary kidney).
  - Acute tubular necrosis (ATN):
    - Prerenal condition.
    - Nephrotoxic medications (antibiotics, chemotherapy).
    - Contrast agents.
    - Hemoglobinuria, myoglobinuria.
    - Tumor lysis syndrome.
  - Microangiopathy.
- Postrenal failure:
  - Intra-abdominal tumors compressing ureters or bladder:
    - Retroperitoneal sarcomas.
    - Lymphomas.
    - Germ cell tumors, stromal ovarian tumors, adrenal or celiac axis neuroblastomas.

Management

- Treatment of the underlying etiology if possible.
- Monitor accurate intake and output, daily weight.
- Administer fluids appropriately:
  - Total fluid intake (TFI) = urine output + insensible losses (400 cc/m2/day in an afebrile child) + other losses if euvolemic.
- Furosemide in fluid-overloaded patients.
- Closely monitor serum urea creatinine, sodium, potassium, chloride, calcium, magnesium phosphate, and total CO_2 and correct metabolic abnormalities.

- Order CT or renal Doppler ultrasound of the abdomen:
  - May use contrast if no evidence of renal failure.
  - If contrast is required, request isotonic contrast (visipaque).
  - Gadolinium is contraindicated with GFR < 60 ml/min/1.73 m^2.
- Avoid use of nephrotoxic drugs: Aminoglycosides, vancomycin, amphotericin-B, NSAIDs.
- Adjust all medication for the degree of renal failure.
- In severe cases, may need renal replacement therapy (dialysis).
- Consultation with pediatric nephrology.

References

Albano EA, Sandler E. Oncological emergencies. In: Altman AJ, ed. *Supportive Care of Children with Cancer: Current Therapy and Guidelines from the Children's Oncology Group*. (3rd ed). Baltimore, MD: Johns Hopkins University Press; 2004:221–242.

Lemaire M, Radhakrishnan S, Licht C. Fluids, electrolytes and acid-base. In: Dipchand, Friedman, Bismilla, Lam, Gupta (eds). *The Hospital for Sick Children Handbook of Pediatrics*. 11th ed. Toronto, ON: Elsevier; 2009: 283–312.

Pizzo PA, Poplack DG, eds. *Principles and Practice of Pediatric Oncology*. 5th ed. Philadelphia, Pa: Lippincott Williams & Wilkins; 2006.

Truong TH, Beyene J, Hitzler J, et al. Features at presentation predict children with acute lymphoblastic leukemia at low risk for tumor lysis syndrome. *Cancer*. 2007;110(8):1832–1839.

chapter   1 7

Thrombotic Emergencies

Leonardo R. Brandao and Suzan Williams

Outline

- Introduction
- Disseminated Intravascular Coagulation
- Thrombotic Events
- Antithrombotic Therapy

Introduction

- *Hemostasis* is the physiologic response of the coagulation system triggered by vessel injury to promote blood flow arrest.
- *Thrombosis* occurs in consequence to an excessive response of the coagulation system, leading to formation of a blood clot inside of a vein/artery, with subsequent partial or complete blood flow obstruction of the affected vessel.

- *Thromboembolism* is the clinical consequence that results from either excessive clot formation (promoted by the coagulation cascade) and/or lack of clot inhibition (promoted by natural anticoagulant pathways), when the clot itself (thrombus) or its fragments are carried by the bloodstream.
- *Thrombotic events (TE)* occur within the superficial (SVT) or deep venous system (DVT), pulmonary vessels (PE), arterial vascular tree, or within the central nervous system.
- Thrombosis is recognized as a major health problem in adults, but it can also affect pediatric patients.
- In patients with cancer, the hemostatic balance is shifted towards excessive thrombus formation, and there are several acquired coagulation-related imbalances with significant clinical consequences.

Disseminated Intravascular Coagulation (DIC)

Definition

- Acquired syndrome of various etiologies characterized by the intravascular activation of coagulation.
- DIC can originate from and cause damage to the microvasculature, which, if severe, can produce organ dysfunction.
- Always secondary to an underlying disorder of a wide variety.
- Among those potential conditions complicated by DIC, acute leukemias and solid tumors (e.g., disseminated rhabdomyosarcomas) have long been described as potential triggers of coagulation derangements in children with cancer.

Pathophysiology

- Consumptive coagulopathy characterized by microscopic thrombi formation within the microcirculation leading to platelet and clotting factor consumption.
- The resulting microangiopathic process, if widespread and severe, can lead to multiple organ dysfunction.
- As DIC progresses, platelet and clotting factor consumption exceeds their production rate and the balance of coagulation and fibrinolysis is disrupted → bleeding (Figure 17-1).

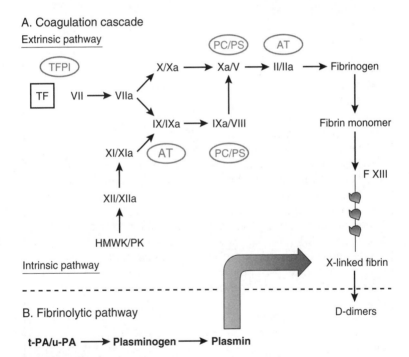

Legend: Gray: natural coagulation inhibitors; Black: procoagulant system; Bold: fibrinolytic pathway

Abbreviations: PC: protein C; PS: protein S; AT: antithrombin; TFPI: tissue factor pathway inhibitor; TF: tissue factor; VII: factor VII; VIIa: activated factor VII; X: factor X; Xa: activated factor X; V: factor V; II: prothrombin; IIa: thrombin; IX: factor IX; IXa: activated factor IX; FXIII: factor XIII; XII: factor XII; XIIa: activated factor XII; HMWK: high molecular weight kininogen; PK: pre-kalikrein; X-linked: crosslinked; t-PA: tissue plasminogen activator; u-PA: urokinase

Figure 17-1 The coagulation cascade and the fibrinolytic pathway.

- Despite the wide variety of precipitating conditions (Table 17-1), the syndrome appears to result from one of two general processes:
  - Induction by a systemic inflammatory response with activation of the cytokine network.

Table 17-1   Disorders associated with DIC relevant to pediatric oncology.

Infectious (cytokine-/inflammatory-mediated)
- Bacterial: Meningococcal, gram-negative microorganisms
- Viral: Herpes, respiratory syncycial respiratory virus
- Protozoan: Malaria
- Other: Candida, aspergillus

Malignancies (inflammatory-mediated, direct coagulation activation, and abnormal fibrinolysis)
- Myeloproliferative conditions
- Leukemias: ALL, AML (monocytic and APL)
- Solid tumors: Disseminated neuroblastoma or rhabdomyosarcoma

Tissue damage (release/exposure of tissue factor)
- Rhabdomyolysis
- Severe asphyxia and/or hypoxia
- Profound hypovolemic/hemorraghic shock

Vascular malformations (abnormal endothelium and blood flow)
- Hemangiomas, kaposiform hemangio-endotheliomas (KMS)
- Venous/venous lymphatic capillary malformation (KTS)

Microangiopathic disorders (abnormal endothelial activation and blood flow)
- Severe thrombotic thrombocytopenia purpura (cyclosporine/BMT-induced)

Immunologic disorders (complement activation and tissue factor release)
- Severe graft rejection
- Severe acute hemolytic transfusion reaction

Others:
- Fulminant hepatic failure
- Acquired protein C deficiency
- Massive blood transfusion

NOTES: ALL, acute lymphoblastic leukemia; AML, acute nonlymphoblastic leukemia; APL, acute promyelocytic leukemia; KMS, Kasabach-Merritt syndrome; KTS, Klippel-Trenaunay syndrome; BMT, bone marrow transplantation

○ Direct activation of coagulation with the release or exposure of procoagulant material into the bloodstream, overwhelming the natural anticoagulant system.

• The specific mechanisms that drive the process, particularly for inflammatory-mediated DIC, can be summarized as follows (Figure 17-2):

1. Activation of coagulation leads to widespread microvascular thrombosis → multiorgan failure secondary

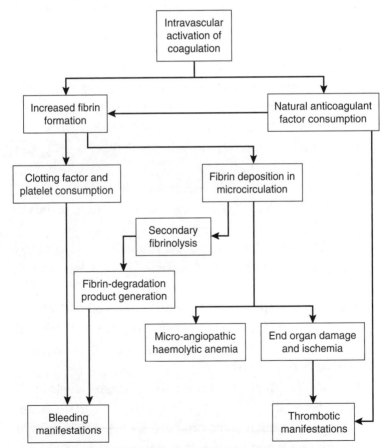

Figure 17-2 Pathophysiology of the clinical manifestations of disseminated intravascular coagulation.

to enhanced fibrin formation and/or decreased fibrin removal.

2. Increased intravascular coagulation is followed by secondary fibrinolysis → consumption of clotting factors and platelets.

3. An increase in the plasma concentration of fibrin degradation products further promotes fibrinolysis.

DIC in Children with Cancer

- Both solid tumors and hematological malignancies may be complicated by DIC.
- Tissue factor (TF) expressed by cancer cells is important in the pathogenesis of DIC.
- Solid tumors can also express other procoagulant molecules such as cancer procoagulant, a cysteine protease with factor X-activating properties.
- Children with acute promyelocytic leukemia (APL) can present with DIC due to:
  - ○ The t(15;17) in APL cells induces hyperexpression of TF in the leukemic cell leading to activation of the coagulation cascade.
  - ○ APL blasts have increased Annexin-II receptor expression, which binds to tissue plasminogen activator leading to increased fibrinolysis.
- Chemotherapy can increase the risk of DIC as antithrombin (AT) levels are decreased due to increased consumption and decreased synthesis (e.g., L-asparaginase formulations).
- In severe infections and sepsis decreased levels of AT precede clinical findings of sepsis, and there is decreased function of the protein C pathway as a result of both decreased levels and down-regulation of thrombomodulin.

Clinical Aspects

- Diverse clinical spectrum ranging from subclinical decrease in the platelet count or prolongation in the clotting times, to fulminant DIC → widespread microvascular thrombosis and profuse bleeding.
- Severe or overt DIC usually manifests as spontaneous ecchymoses, petechiae, purpura, trauma- or procedure-related oozing, or spontaneous bleeding.
- Purpura fulminans is present only in case of severe protein C depletion, but mild microangiopathic hemolytic anemia is frequently noted in association with widespread metastatic malignancy.

Table 17-2 Diagnostic scoring system for overt DIC.

Global coagulation test results	Score (0, 1, or 2 points)
Platelet count	$> 100 \times 10^9/l = 0$
	$50 - 100 \times 10^9/l = 1$
	$< 50 \times 10^9/l = 2$
Elevated fibrin-related markers	No increase = 0
(soluble fibrin monomers; D-dimers	Moderated increase = 1
fibrin/fibrinogen degradation products)	Strong increase = 2
Prolonged prothrombin time	< 3 sec = 0
(in seconds [sec] above upper limit of normal)	3–6 sec = 1
	> 6 sec = 2
Fibrinogen level	> 1.0 g/l = 0
	< 1.0 g/l = 1
TOTAL SCORE =	

If score ≥ 5, compatible with overt DIC, recommended repeating score daily.
If score < 5, suggestive (not affirmative) for nonovert DIC, repeat scoring in 1–2 days.
Source: Taylor FB Jr, Toh CH, Hoots WK, Wada H, Levi M. Towards definition, clinical and laboratory criteria, and a scoring system for disseminated coagulation. *Thromb Haemost.* 2001;86:1327–1330.

- In pediatric oncology, sepsis is one of the most common etiologies of DIC:
  - There is no difference in the incidence of DIC between gram-negative or gram-positive organisms, suggesting DIC is triggered either by specific components from the microorganism cell membrane (lipopolyssacharide or endotoxin) or bacterial exotoxins (e.g., staphylococcal alpha toxin).

Diagnosis

The diagnosis of DIC cannot be established on the basis of a single laboratory test, but requires assessment of the entire clinical picture.

- Helpful tests for diagnosis of DIC include:
  - Complete blood count and smear: Rule out thrombocytopenia and/or fragmented red cells.
  - Prothrombin time/international normalized ratio (PT/INR).
  - Activated partial thromboplastin time (aPTT).
  - D-dimer.
  - Fibrinogen-degradation products (FDPs).
  - Fibrinogen level.
- Interpretation of all coagulation-related laboratory results always requires proper assessment by comparison with age-appropriate normal reference values.

Treatment

- Aggressive treatment of the underlying condition and supportive care.
- Volume resuscitation, inotropic/vasopressor support, antimicrobials, and respiratory support as needed.
- Plasma/platelet substitution should be used in patients with active bleeding, those undergoing an invasive

procedure, or those with a significant depletion of these hemostatic factors.

- Maintain the platelet count > 30 to $50 \times 10^9/l$ in non-critical patients, and fibrinogen $> 1 g/l$.

- Clotting factors can be replaced by either frozen plasma (FFP), which provides all coagulation and anti-coagulation factors, administered every 12 to 24 hours at a dose of 10–20 ml/kg per infusion; or by cryoprecipitate, which has a higher concentration of von Willebrand's factor, fibrinogen, factor XIII, and factor VIII.

- Cryoprecipitate is used for correction of hypofibrinogenemia (1 bag per 5 kg of body weight) and can be administered every 6 to 12 hours.

- For catastrophic nonresponsive bleeding, judicious use of recombinant activated factor VII (rFVIIa) should be instituted with the help of an experienced hematologist.

- No beneficial effect of anticoagulant therapy with full-dose heparin. Use of low-dose heparin is warranted in a case-by-case basis.

- The administration of AT and activated protein C concentrate remains controversial. While the former may have utility in severe AT depletion secondary to chemotherapy-induced DIC in pediatric ALL (50 to 200 units/kg/dose), the latter may be considered in cases of severe sepsis or in cases of purpura fulminans. In both cases, a consultation with a pediatric hematologist is strongly recommended.

Thrombotic Events

Introduction

- Procoagulant mechanisms and natural anticoagulant inhibitors are intrinsically related in a delicate equilibrium. This can be disrupted by an inherited or acquired condition leading to excessive prothrombotic stimuli or lack of proper coagulation inhibition.

- Thrombin is the most powerful procoagulant protein that promotes the formation of a stable clot.
- The natural anticoagulant systems (e.g., AT, protein C/S system) together with the endothelial (i.e., heparin cofactor II) and the fibrinolytic system act as a counterbalance to clot formation.
- The hemostatic system in infants and children is significantly different than in adults, with many of the hemostatic components present in different concentrations; therefore, children respond to anticoagulant and thrombolytic therapy differently than adults.

Epidemiology

- Venous thromboembolism (VTE) is being diagnosed with increasing frequency in children.
- Incidence: 0.7–1.9 per 100,000.
- Morbidity: Recurrent thrombosis (21%), postphlebitic syndrome (7–70%); clinically significant postphlebitic syndrome (10–15%).
- Mortality: thrombosis-specific (2–7%).
- Age distribution of pediatric VTE appears as a bimodal curve, with the highest incidence in:
  - Neonates, due to lower concentration of coagulation inhibitors (AT, protein C/S, heparin cofactor-II) and decreased fibrinolytic capacity.
  - Adolescents, due to increased capacity for thrombin generation, a new decrease in the fibrinolytic system, and an increase in acquired risk factors (e.g., smoking, pregnancy, use of oral contraceptives, and obesity).
- The rate of VTE in blacks is twice that of whites in the United States for children of all age groups.

Etiology

- Diverse and multifactorial in approximately 75 % of children diagnosed with VTE.
- Genetic and acquired factors contribute to TE in children.
- Clinical conditions: Malignancies (mostly ALL), congenital heart disease, trauma, renal disease and infections.
- Drugs: L-asparaginase, oral contraceptives.
- Surgery.

Thrombosis and Cancer in Children

- The reported incidence of VTE in childhood ALL varies from 1.1 % to 36.7 %, with an overall average of 5 %.
- In patients with lymphomas, solid tumors, and brain tumors, the estimated incidence of symptomatic TE is approximately 7–16 %.
- In the Canadian Pediatric Thrombophilia Registry, 25 % of patients were diagnosed with cancer, and 40 % had a central venous line.
- TE in children with malignancies occurs in order of decreasing frequency: ALL, sarcomas, lymphomas, AML, Wilms' tumor, neuroblastomas, and brain tumors.
- Risk factors in ALL include presence of a CVL; chemotherapy regimens containing L-asparaginase in combination with steroids; older age; high-risk disease, and probably inherited thrombophilia. For sarcomas (rhabdomyosarcomas > Ewing's > osteosarcomas) risk factors include advanced disease staging and tumor location. For lymphomas, risk factors include age (> 10 years), advanced stage, and mediastinal mass.
- *CVL-related thrombosis*:
  - CVLs are the most common risk factor for TE in children with cancer.

- ○ Incidence: 0–50% depending on study design, diagnostic methods used, type of malignancy, and treatment protocols.
- ○ Predisposing factors:
  - ■ Damage to the vessel wall during insertion.
  - ■ Vein accessed—left > right side.
  - ■ Location of the catheter—femoral > brachiocephalic > jugular.
  - ■ Large bore catheter use in relatively small vessels.
  - ■ Catheter material.
  - ■ Duration of catheter stay.
  - ■ Content of the infusate, e.g., TPN.
- ○ Symptoms:
  - ■ Inability to aspirate from or infuse blood through catheter.
  - ■ Recurrent bacteremias.
  - ■ Swelling and/or redness within the extremity/region where catheter is located.
  - ■ Superior vena cava syndrome: Pain, swelling, collateral vessel formation, chylothorax, and/or symptoms of pulmonary embolus.
- • Studies where venography was systematically used reported incidence rates between 37.6% (PARKAA Study; ALL) and 50% (ALL and non-ALL cases). Studies where ultrasound or echocardiograms were obtained only if a clinical suspicion for TE occurrence was present documented the lowest incidence rates (0% to 8.8%).

Clinical Presentations

- • Thrombotic events can present in the venous or arterial territory. Most commonly, venous events encompass the deep venous system (DVT) or pulmonary vessels

(PE). They can also present in the brain, as cerebral sinus venous thrombosis (CSVT) or as arterial ischemic infarcts (AIS).

- Most commonly, ALL is associated with DVTs or CSVTs (CSVT corresponds to approximately 50% of TE in children with ALL). Similarly, solid tumors are also associated most commonly with DVTs.
- Emergencies usually take place secondary to complete obstruction of the superior vena cava (SVC syndrome), bilateral PEs, CSVTs, acute arterial ischemic limbs or, more rarely, intracardiac thrombotic events.
- DVT presents with limb swelling, color change (bluish-reddish), increased temperature, pain, and edema.
- PE presents with chest pain, shortness of breath, hemoptysis, and pleuritic pain.
- CSVT in infants usually presents as seizures (e.g., generalized); in older children, CVST presents with neurological local findings (e.g., hemiparesis, abnormal cranial nerve findings).
- Arterial events present as cold, ischemic, painful, pale limbs or with affected extremities where pain is triggered by exertion and/or limb movement.
- Intracardiac events present with weakness, shortness of breath, intolerance to exertion, chest pain, or loss of consciousness.

Antithrombotic Therapy

- Pediatric patients diagnosed with DVTs, PEs, arterial events, and CSVTs are usually treated with one of three commonly used anticoagulants agents (Tables 17-3 through 17-6). Fibrinolytic therapy is indicated when life, limb, or organ are at risk.

Text continued on page 304

Table 17-3 Unfractionated heparin dosing.

Loading dose: 50–75 units/kg, IV, over 10 minutes

Maintenance dose: ≤ 1 year of age: 28 units/kg/h

> 1 year of age: 20 units/kg/h

aPTT (seconds)	Anti-Xa (units/ml)	Bolus (Units/kg)	HOLD (minutes)	Rate Change	Repeat aPTT
< 50	< 0.1	50	0	Increase 10%	4 hours
50–59	0.1–0.34	0	0	Increase 10%	4 hours
60–85	0.35–0.7	0	0	0	24 hours
86–95	0.71–0.89	0	0	Decrease 10%	4 hours
96–120	0.9–1.20	0	30	Decrease 10%	4 hours
> 120	> 1.20	0	60	Decrease 10%	4 hours

Adapted from: Taylor FB Jr, Toh CH, Hoots WK, Wada H, Levi M. Towards definition, clinical and laboratory criteria, and a scoring system for disseminated coagulation. Thromb Haemost 2001; 86: 1327–1330.

Table 17-4 Low molecular weight (LMWH – enoxaparin) dosing.

	Age ≤ 2 months	Age > 2 months to 18 years
Initial treatment dose	1.75 mg/kg/dose SC q 12 h	1 mg/kg/dose SQ q 12 h
Initial prophylactic dose	0.75 mg/kg/dose SC q 12 h or 1.5 mg/kg/dose SQ q 24 h	0.5 mg/kg/dose SQ q 12 h or 1 mg/kg/dose SC q 24 h

Table 17-5 Low molecular weight (LMWH – enoxaparin) adjustment.

Anti-Xa (units/kg)	HOLD	Dose Change	Repeat Anti-Xa
< 0.35	No	Increase 25%	4 hours post next dose
0.35–0.49	No	Increase 10%	4 hours post next dose
0.5–1.0	No	0	1 × wk; 4 hours post morning dose
1.01–1.5	No	Decrease 20%	4 hours post morning dose
1.6–2.0	3 hours	Decrease 30%	Trough level prior to next dose; and then 4 hours post morning dose
> 2.0	Yes (until level < 0.5)	Decrease 40%	Trough level prior to next dose, until level < 0.5, and then 4 hours post morning dose

Table 17-6 Warfarin loading doses (days 2–4).
Loading dose: 0.2 mg/kg PO, q day; maximum 5 mg
0.1 mg/kg; with liver dysfunction, Fontan
procedure, or severe renal impairment

INR	1.1–1.3	Repeat initial loading dose
INR	1.4–3.0	50% of initial loading dose
INR	3.1–3.5	25% of initial loading dose
INR	> 3.5	Hold until INR < 3.5, then restart at 50% less than previous dose

Adapted from: Taylor FB Jr, Toh CH, Hoots WK, Wada H, Levi M. Towards definition, clinical and laboratory criteria, and a scoring system for disseminated coagulation. Thromb Haemost 2001; 86: 1327-30.

- For PEs, fibrinolysis should only be used if cardiovascular imbalance is present.

- *Unfractionated heparin (UFH) and low-molecular weight heparin (LMWH)*: Both agents differ in terms of their molecular weight and mechanism of action. Standard heparin (UFH), the longer molecule, has a shorter half-life (30 to 60 minutes), and its effects can be immediately and completely reversed by protamine sulphate. Heparin binds to the natural anticoagulant antithrombin (AT) and increases the rate of inhibition of activated factors II (IIa) and X (Xa). Because of its bigger molecular weight, UFH binds nonspecifically to other molecules, resulting in a less predictable response. Its anticoagulation activity can be monitored in the laboratory by either the activated partial thromboplastin time (aPTT) or by the anti-Xa assay. The incidence of major bleeding associated with UFH is approximately 12%.

- The advantages of low-molecular weight heparin (LMWH) in relation to UFH include higher bioavailability; prompt anticoagulation activity; lack of necessity for intravenous access and for daily laboratory monitoring; and lower risks of bleeding, drug-induced osteopenia, and heparin-induced thrombocytopenia. LMWH possess a longer half-life and higher specific anti-Xa activity, being less dependent on its interaction with AT. Laboratory monitoring, achieved by the anti-Xa assay, is required in children, especially if decreased renal function (e.g., post-cisplatin) is present. There are several forms of LMWH available (e.g., enoxaparin, reviparin, tinzaparin, dalteparin), and the formulation most commonly used in children is *enoxaparin*. A proposed dose-adjustment algorithm for both agents is included in Table 17-3. With this drug, minor and major bleeding occurs at approximately 25% and 5%, respectively. In addition, temporary hair loss, elevated liver enzymes, heparin-induced thrombocytopenia, and osteopenia have also been described in children.

- *Vitamin K antagonists*: Warfarin exerts its anticoagulant power by reduction of functional circulating levels of vitamin-K-dependent (VKDF) factors II, VII, IX, and X, via inhibition of their γ-carboxylation. Its laboratory monitoring is achieved by blood sampling for PT/INR, with target ranges similar to the ones used in the adult population. The different half-lives (6 to 60 hours) and physiologically distinct age-dependent VKDF levels contribute to a less predictive response to this agent. Its use can be challenging, as it is also affected by multiple medications and diet (infant formula is supplemented with vitamin K in North America). Warfarin has been classically utilized for both primary (e.g., mechanical heart valves) and for secondary thromboprophylaxis (e.g., deep vein thrombosis/pulmonary embolism). Bleeding is its most feared and frequent complication, as major bleeding events occur at a rate of 0.5% per patient-year in children, with an overall incidence of 12%. More rarely, hair loss, osteopenia, tracheal calcification, and teratogenicity have also been described. It is very important to ensure appropriate patient education to all children/families receiving this agent.

- *Fibrinolytic therapy*: The most common agent currently utilized is tPA. This agent can be infused locally (0.04 mg/kg/hour), when a multifenestrated catheter has its tip inserted as close as possible to the thrombus site, or it can be administered systemically. For the latter option, systemic courses are divided into low-dose (0.01–0.06 mg/kg/hour) or normal/high-dose (0.1–0.6 mg/kg/hour, over 6 hours). At the end of each course, repeated imaging for objective documentation of clot response (decrease in clot size) is recommended. For neonates, a head ultrasound prior to fibrinolytic therapy is suggested, to rule out intracranial bleeding. In case the decision is in favor of tPA infusion, fresh frozen plasma (FFP) (10–20 ml/kg) is also recommended, due to age-appropriate response differences. The incidence of major bleeding ranges from 5% to 10%.
- *Blocked central venous lines*: see Chapter 19.

References

Andrew M, Paes B, Milner R, Johnston M, Mitchell L, Tollefsen DM, Powers P. Development of the human coagulation system in the full-term infant. *Blood*. 1987;70:165–172.

Athale U, Siciliano S, Thabane L, et al. Epidemiology and clinical risk factors predisposing to thromboembolism in children with cancer. *Pediatr Blood Cancer*. 2008;51:792–797.

Caruso V, Iacoviello L, Castelnuovo AD, et al. Thrombotic complications in childhood acute lymphoblastic leukemia: a meta-analysis of 17 prospective studies comprising 1752 pediatric patients. *Blood*. 2006;108:2216–2222.

Falanga A, Rickles FR. Management of thrombohemorraghic syndrome in hematologic malignancies. *Hematol Am Soc Hematol Educ Program*. 2007;2007:165–171.

Mitchell LG, Halton JM, Vegh PA, et al. Effect of disease and chemotherapy inducing high dose methylprednisolone and L-asparaginase. *Leuk Lymphoma*. 1999;33:361–364.

Monagle P, Adams M, Mahoney M, et al. Outcome of pediatric thromboembolic disease: a report from the Canadian Childhood Thrombophilia Registry. *Pediatr Res*. 2000;47:763–766.

Monagle P, Barnes C, Ignjatovic V, et al. Developmental haemostasis. Impact for clinical haemostasis laboratories. *Thromb Haemost*. 2006;95:362–372.

Ribeiro R, Pui C. The clinical and biological correlates of coagulopathy in children with acute leukemia. *J Clin Oncol*. 1986;4:1212–1218.

c h a p t e r   1 8

The Basics of Chemotherapy

Vicky R. Breakey, Tony H.Truong, and Angela Punnett

Outline

- Mechanism of Action
- Side Effects of Chemotherapy
- Specific Chemotherapeutic Agents: Mechanisms, Pharmacology, and Selected Toxicities
- Interactions Between Methotrexate and Selected Commonly Used Drugs

Mechanism of Action

- Target vital molecules or metabolic pathways.
- Most target DNA, RNA, or protein synthesis and function.
- Nonselective: Damages cancer cells and normal cells.

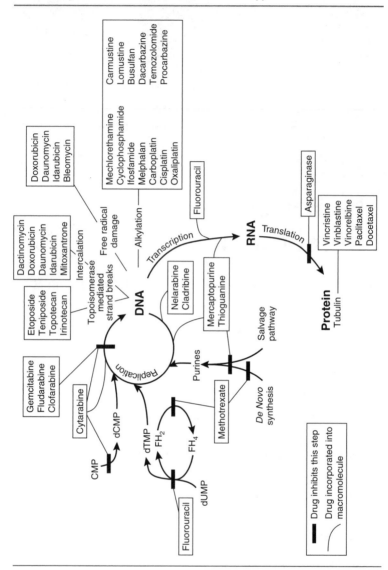

Figure 18-1 Site of action of commonly used anti-cancer drugs. CMP, cytidine monophosphate; dCMP, deoxycytidine monophosphate; dTMP, deoxythymidine monophosphate; dUMP, deoxyuridine monophosphate; FH2, dihydrofolate; FH4, tetrahydropholate.

Courtesy of Adamson PC, Balis FM, Berg S, Blaney SM. General Principles of Chemotherapy. In: Pizzo PA, Poplack DG, ed. *Principles and Practice of Pediatric Oncology*, 5th ed. Philadelphia: Lippincott Williams & Wilkins, 2006; 294.

- Normal cells are able to monitor and repair damaged DNA, except after very high doses of chemotherapy.
- See Figure 18-1 for illustration of site of action for common antineoplastic agents.

Classes of Anticancer Drugs

- Antimetabolites.
- Alkylating agents.
- Antitumor antibiotics.
- Plant products.
- Miscellaneous agents.
- Biologic agents.
- Hormonal agents.
- Novel therapies.

Side Effects of Chemotherapy

- Each drug has a unique side effect profile (see following tables).
- Side effects common to many drugs include:
  - Fatigue.
  - Nausea/vomiting.
  - Mucositis.
  - Skin rash.
  - Hair loss.
  - Bone marrow suppression.
- Two side effects that deserve special mention:
  - Infertility (particularly with alkylators).
  - Second malignancy (particularly with epipodophyllotoxins, alkylators, anthracyclines).

- *Extravasation:*
  - Chemotherapy drugs are characterized as nonvesicants, irritants, or vesicants.
  - Refer to institutional policies for tactics to prevent extravasation and for specific management in the event of extravasation.
  - Irritants:
    - May cause pain and phlebitis at injection site.
    - With extravasation: local treatment with hot or cold compresses may decrease symptoms.
    - Sclerosis and hyperpigmentation along the vein usually resolve without sequelae.
  - Vesicants:
    - May cause progressive tissue damage at injection site.
    - Extravasation from a peripheral IV (PIV) may cause pain, erythema, soft tissue damage, with or without necrosis.
    - Extravasation from central catheter may result in erythema, soft tissue damage, with or without necrosis, and potential structural damage.

Text continued on page 328

Table 18-1 Chemotherapeutic Agents: Alkylators.

Drug	Mechanism and Pharmacology	Vesicant?	Selected Toxicities (A, E, D, L)*
Busulfan	• Alkylates DNA, leading to breaks in the DNA molecule and cross-linking of DNA strands, interferes with DNA replication and RNA transcription • Hepatic metabolism, urinary excretion	YES	• A: allergic reaction, tachycardia, tamponade, hypertension • E: electrolyte disturbances, renal dysfunction, veno-occlusive disease, rash • D: hyperpigmentation, cholestatic hepatitis • L: secondary leukemia, delayed puberty, early menopause, infertility
Carboplatin	• Analog of cisplatin, more stable • Renal excretion	No	• Similar to cisplatin, but less nephrotoxicity, neurotoxicity, ototoxicity, and emetogenesis • Hypersensitivity is more common than for cisplatin
Carmustine (BCNU)	• Alkylates DNA and RNA, can cross-link DNA, and inhibits several enzymes by carbamoylation • Highly lipid soluble, crosses blood-brain barrier • Metabolized by liver, excretion via kidneys and lungs (10%) • Also used as implantable wafer in CNS tumors	No (irritant)	• A: N/V • E: myelosuppression, hepatotoxicity (up to 60 d post), early onset pneumonitis, ocular toxicities, ataxia/dizziness/encephalopathy • L: secondary malignancies, infertility, late onset pneumonitis

(continued)

Table 18-1 (continued).

Drug	Mechanism and Pharmacology	Vesicant?	Selected Toxicities (A, E, D, L)*
Cisplatin	• Intracellular activation forms reactive platinum complexes that inhibit DNA synthesis by forming cross-linking of DNA • Renal excretion	No (irritant)	• A: hypersensitivity, N/V, electrolyte disturbances • E: ototoxicity, myelosuppression, neurotoxicity, nephrotoxicity • D: delayed N/V • L: secondary leukemia
Cyclophosphamide	• Cross-links strands of DNA and RNA and inhibits protein synthesis • Metabolized mainly in the liver; cytochrome P450 • Limited crossing of blood-brain barrier (BBB) • Excreted in the urine	No	• A: anaphylaxis, facial flushing, nasal congestion, headache • E: myelosuppression, hyperpigmentation, anorexia, N/V, diarrhea, mucositis, hemmorrhagic cystitis (up to 40%) • D: cardiac dysfunction (high doses), pneumonitis, renal tubular necrosis, gonadal suppression/amennorrhea, SIADH • L: pulmonary fibrosis (weeks-months), secondary malignancies (bladder, myeloproliferative, lymphoproliferative, infertility

Dacarbazine	• Activated in the liver to methyltriazenoimi-dazole carboxamide (MTIC) • MTIC forms methylcarbonium ions that attach nucleophilic groups in DNA • Primarily renal excretion, some hepatobiliary and pulmonary	No (irritant)	• A: N/V, rare anaphylaxis • E: myelosuppression • E/D: hepatotoxicity with hepatic necrosis and/or hepatic vascular occlusion
Ifosfamide	• Structural analogue of cyclophosphamide (mechanism of action presumed to be identical) • Metabolized by liver, excreted by kidneys	No	• A: N/V, encephalopathy (confusion, lethargy, somnolence, seizures, coma, onset 2 h to 28 days postinfusion), SIADH, metabolic acidosis (30%), hemmorrhagic cystitis • E: myelosuppression, immunosuppression, arrhythmia (at high doses) • D: pneumonitis (interstitial, rare) • L: gonadal damage, sterility, proximal tubular damage
Lomustine (CCNU)	• Alkylates DNA and RNA, can cross-link DNA, and inhibits several enzymes by carbamoylation • Rapidly absorbed • Readily passes BBB • Metabolized by liver, excreted by kidney and lung (10%)	No	• A: N/V • D: myelosuppression is cumulative and often starts 4–6 weeks after administration • L: pulmonary fibrosis (6 m to 15 y after therapy)

(continued)

Table 18-1 (continued).

Drug	Mechanism and Pharmacology	Vesicant?	Selected Toxicities (A, E, D, L)*
Mechlorethamine (Nitrogen Mustard)	• Interferes with DNA replication and RNA transcription as the result of formation of unstable carbonium ions that cross-link with DNA • Metabolized by rapid hydrolysis by body fluids and demethylation in liver • Combines with water or reactive cell compounds and is undetectable in the blood within minutes	YES	• A: anticholinergic effect, anaphylaxis, neurotoxicity • E: N/V, myelosuppression, mucositis • D: ototoxicity, neurotoxicity, nausea/vomiting, ammenorrhea, sclerosing thrombophlebitis (1–10%) • L: secondary malignancies (1–6%), infertility
Melphalan	• L-isomer of mechlorethamine (see above) • Inhibits DNA and RNA synthesis by cross-linking with DNA • Not actively metabolized, hydrolyzed spontaneously, some hepatic conjugation	YES	• A: anaphylaxis, N/V, diarrhea (usually 1 week post) • E: cytopenias, immunosuppression • D: pulmonary fibrosis, interstitial pneumonitis • L: secondary leukemia, carcinoma, myeloproliferative syndrome

| Procarbazine | • Derivative of hydrazine whose mechanism of action has not yet been clearly defined
• MAO inhibiting properties (N.B. avoid foods rich in tyramine to avoid interactions, tyramine syndrome)
• Primarily hepatic excretion, some renal and pulmonary | No | • A: allergic reaction, N/V
• E: bone marrow suppression, rash, bleeding, hypertension
• E/D: hepatotoxicity, pancreatitis, thrombosis, pulmonary toxicity
• L: secondary malignancies, infertility |
| Temozolomide | • Rapid chemical conversion at physiologic pH to the MTIC (see mechanism for decarbazine)
• Rapid oral absorption, 100 % bioavailability | No | • A: N/V, headache, decreased LOC/amnesia, seizure (3 %), pain, myalgia
• E: myelosuppression, fatigue, anorexia, fever, diarrhea, constipation, dyspnea, bleeding, thrombosis, neuropathy
• D, L: ovarian suppression, infertility |

NOTE: Toxicities: A = acute (time of infusion—minutes to days), E = early (days to weeks), D = delayed (during course of therapy—weeks to months), L = late (months to years posttreatment) N/V = nausea and vomiting.

Table 18-2 Chemotherapeutic Agents: Antimetabolites.

Drug	Mechanism and Pharmacology	Vesicant?	Selected Toxicities (A, E, D, L)*
Cladribine	• Synthetic purine nucleoside prodrug, resistant to deamination by adenosine deaminase resulting in intracellular accumulation • Incorporates, preventing elongation	No	• A: constitutional symptoms, rash • E: severe myelosuppression, immunosuppression • D: neurotoxicity (high dose), renal insufficiency
Clofarabine	• Purine nucleoside analog • Inhibits DNA repair and synthesis of DNA and RNA, induces apoptosis	No	• A: N/V, diarrhea, tachycardia, severe inflammatory response syndrome (SIRS) (rare). • E: myelosuppression, hepato-biliary toxicities, pericardial effusion
Cytarabine (Ara-C)	• Pyrimidine analog—resembles cytidine • Hepatic metabolism	No	• E: pancytopenia, fever (> 80%), bowel necrosis, NEC, severe rash (< 1%), conjunctivitis • E/D: Neurotoxicity • A/E: *Cytarabine syndrome*, a flulike syndrome, characterized by fever, myalgia, bone pain, maculopapular rash, conjunctivitis, malaise, and occasionally chest pain, may begin 6–12 h after IV cytarabine, occurs more commonly after large doses

Fludarabine	• Synthetic analog of the purine nucleoside antiviral agent vidarabine • Inhibits DNA replication enzymes and is incorporated as a false nucleoside to inhibit elongation • Active in the S-phase of cell division excreted in the urine	No	• A: anaphylaxis, constitutional symptoms, diarrhea • E: myelosuppression, GI bleeding, autoimmune hemolytic anemia and neutropenia; ITP • D: neurotoxicity, pneumonitis/pulmonary fibrosis
5-Fluorouracil (5-FU)	• Pyrimidine analog—resembles uracil • Hepatic metabolism	No	• E: pancytopenia, cardiac arrhythmia, diarrhea, stomatitis • E: Palmar-plantar dysesthesia (hand and foot syndrome)
Gemcitabine	• A pyrimidine analog, similar to cytarabine, but with a wider spectrum of antitumor activity • Inhibits DNA synthesis and induces apoptosis • Cell-cycle phase specific (S and G_1/S-phases) • Metabolites excreted in urine	No	• A: anaphylaxis, N/V, diarrhea, constitutional symptoms, rash, dyspnea • E: myelosuppression, transaminitis, edema • D: peripheral neuropathy, pulmonary toxicity, hemolytic uremic syndrome (rare)
Mercaptopurine (6-MP)	• Purine analog—resembles hypoxanthine • Hepatic metabolism	No	• E: rash, pancytopenia, stomatitis, oral lesions resembling thrush • E/D: hepatotoxicity (30%), elevated LFTs

(continued)

Table 18-2 (continued).

Drug	Mechanism and Pharmacology	Vesicant?	Selected Toxicities (A, E, D, L)*
Methotrexate (MTX)	• Folate analog—resembles folic acid • Hepatic metabolism • May accumulate in 3rd spaces • Good CNS penetration at high doses • Somatic cells rescued by leucovorin calcium • Glucarpidase (carboxypeptidase-G2) hydrolyses methotrexate; used after overdose or when methotrexate clearance is severely impaired • Drug interactions are common—see Table 18-6	No	• A: elevated LFTs, anaphylaxis, fever, chills • E: pancytopenia, stomatitis • E/D: hepatotoxicity, azotemia (HD MTX) • E/L: neurotoxicity (IT), pulmonary toxicity (2–8%)
Nelarabine	• Nucleoside analog that is rapidly converted by cells of lymphoid lineage to its corresponding arabinosylguanine nucleotide triphosphate (araGTP) • Incorporated into the DNA, resulting in inhibition of DNA synthesis and subsequent cytotoxicity	No	• A: constitutional symptoms, N/V, diarrhea • E: myelosuppression, neurotoxicity (decreased level of consciousness, seizure, ataxia coma) • D: neurotoxicity
Thioguanine (6-TG)	• Purine analog—resembles guanine • Hepatic metabolism	No	• E: rash, pancytopenia, stomatitis, oral lesions resembling thrush • E/D: hepatic fibrosis, elevated LFTs

NOTE: Toxicities: A = acute (time of infusion—minutes to days), E = early (days to weeks), D = delayed (during course of

Table 18-3 Chemotherapeutic Agents: Antitumor Antibiotics.

Drug	Mechanism and Pharmacology	Vesicant?	Selected Toxicities (A, E, D, L)*
Bleomycin	• Free radical formation causes DNA strand breaks • Results in inhibition of DNA, RNA, and protein synthesis	No	• A: high fever, chills, rash, idiosyncratic reaction (fever, hypotension, wheezing) • E: mild myelosuppression • E: dermatologic effects: erythema, rash, striae, 2–4 weeks after • D: pneumonitis, pulmonary fibrosis
Dactinomycin	• Intercalation between DNA base pairs results in uncoiling of the helix, inhibiting DNA, RNA, and protein synthesis • Topoisomerase II inhibition resulting in DNA strand breaks • Metabolized in liver	YES	• E: severe diarrhea, stomatitis, myelosuppression, hepatotoxicity • Radiation recall reaction—may increase toxicity of radiotherapy
Doxorubicin Daunomycin Idarubicin	• Intercalation between DNA base pairs results in uncoiling of the helix, inhibiting DNA, RNA, and protein synthesis • Topoisomerase II inhibition results in DNA strand breaks • Free radical formation • Metabolized in liver and excreted in biliary tree • Cardioprotective agent: dezraxozane	YES	• A: fever, chills, rash, arrhythmia, red colored urine, tears • E: pancytopenia, stomatitis, myocarditis-pericarditis syndrome • D/L: cardiomyopathy, congestive heart failure, second malignancy

(continued)

Table 18-3 (continued).

Drug	Mechanism and Pharmacology	Vesicant?	Selected Toxicities (A, E, D, L)*
Mitoxantrone	• Intercalation between DNA base pairs results in uncoiling of the helix, inhibiting DNA, RNA, and protein synthesis • Topoisomerase II inhibition resulting in DNA strand breaks • No free radical formation	No	• A: anaphylaxis, arrhythmia, bluish discoloration of sclera, fingernails, urine • E: myelosuppression, mucositis • D: cardiotoxicity

NOTE: Toxicities: A = acute (time of infusion—minutes to days), E = early (days to weeks), D = delayed (during course of therapy—weeks to months), L = late (months to years posttreatment) N/V = nausea and vomiting

Table 18-4   Chemotherapeutic Agents: Plant Products.

Drug	Mechanism and Pharmacology	Vesicant?	Selected Toxicities (A, E, D, L)*
Etoposide	• Inhibits topoisomerase II, inducing DNA strand breaks and inhibiting DNA synthesis		• A: anaphylaxis, hypotension • E: myelosuppression, fatigue, diarrhea, mucositis, taste alteration • L: secondary leukemia (AML)
Irinotecan Topotecan	• Inhibits topoisomerase I, inducing DNA strand breaks • Primarily hepatic, rapidly converted to SN-38 by hepatic carboxylesterase enzymes • Irinotecan and SN-38 undergo reversible, pH-dependent conversion between the active lactone (acidic pH) and inactive hydroxyacid (basic pH) forms		• E: myelosuppression, mucositis, increased LFTs, insomnia, dizziness • A: acute irinotecan-diarrhea, cholinergic syndrome—both treated with atropine • E: late onset diarrhea (treated with loperamide), pulmonary syndrome of dyspnea, cough, CXR infiltrates • L: secondary leukemia
Teniposide	• Inhibits topoisomerase I, inducing DNA strand breaks • 30–40% absorbed orally • Undergoes reversible, pH-dependent hydrolysis of the active lactone moiety to the inactive hydroxyacid (carboxylate) form		• E: myelosuppression, elevated LFTs, elevated bilirubin, athralgia, myalgia radiation sensitizing agent • L: secondary leukemia

(continued)

Table 18-4 (continued).

Drug	Mechanism and Pharmacology	Vesicant?	Selected Toxicities (A, E, D, L)*
Vincristine/ Vinblastine/ Vinorelbine	• Inhibits microtubule polymerization as well as inducing depolymerization of formed tubules • Block mitosis by arresting cells in the metaphase • Vinca alkaloids are cell cycle phase-specific for M phase and S phase • Metabolized by hepatic cytochrome P450-3A	YES	• A: peripheral neuropathy, jaw pain, headache • E: constipation, abdominal pain, weakness, ptosis, paralytic ileus, SIADH • D: foot drop, loss of DTR, paresthesia myelosuppression is rare

NOTE: Toxicities: A = acute (time of infusion—minutes to days), E = early (days to weeks), D = delayed (during course of therapy—weeks to months), L = late (months to years posttreatment) N/V = nausea and vomiting

Table 18-5 Chemotherapeutic Agents: Miscellaneous.

Drug	Mechanism and Pharmacology	Vesicant?	Selected Toxicities (A, E, D, L)*
ATRA (All trans-retinoic acid)	• Binds to the fusion protein of the t(15;17) (PML/RARA fusion protein) • Induces terminal differentiation of myeloblasts • Metabolized by hepatic cytochrome P450 • Well absorbed with 50% bioavailability	N/A	• E: headache, hyperhistaminemia, ototoxicity, hyperleukocytosis, fatigue, fever, weight gain, cheilitis, skin dryness, rash, elevated LFTs, high triglycerides, high cholesterol, pseudotumor cerebri • E: ATRA syndrome—fever, dyspnea, hypotension, bone pain, respiratory distress, pulmonary infiltrates, hyperleukocytosis, pleural or pericardial effusion, weight gain, lower extremity edema, congestive heart failure, renal failure, and multiorgan failure. Occurs 7–12 days after ATRA. Tx: dexamethasone • E/D: Sweet's syndrome—a hyperinflammatory reaction of neutrophil infiltration of the skin and internal organs, fever, painful erythematous cutaneous plaques—treatment with steroids

(continued)

Table 18-5 (continued).

Drug	Mechanism and Pharmacology	Vesicant?	Selected Toxicities (A, E, D, L)*
Asparaginase	• There are three asparaginases available: E.coli L-asparaginase (from *E. coli*), Erwinia L-asparaginase (isolated from *Erwinia chrysanthem*) and Peg-L-asparaginase (from *E.coli* and attached to polyethylene glycol) • Hydrolyzes the amino acid L-asparagine to L-aspartic acid and ammonia • Asparagine is required for DNA synthesis and cell survival • Most cells are capable of synthesizing asparagine from glutamine but acute lymphoblastic leukemia (ALL) cells lack adequate levels of the required enzyme, asparagine synthetase, and cannot survive asparagine depletion. • Cycle-specific for the G1 phase • Metabolism is unknown, and excretion is possible via reticuloendothelial system.	No	• A: hypersensitivity reactions/anaphylaxis is very common (up to 35%, less for Peg)* • A, E: coagulopathy up to 30% with hypo-fibrinogenemia (> 10%), thrombosis (4% for Peg), pancreatitis (15%), transient hy-perbili (> 10%), transaminitis (> 10%), hepatotoxicity (1–5% for Peg, neurotoxic-ity (> 10%)

Corticosteroids	Cytotoxic to leukemia, myeloma, and lymphoma cells, probably via induction of apoptosis. Specific cellular mechanisms that act to halt DNA synthesis are thought to be related to inhibition of glucose transport or phosphorylation, retardation of mitosis, and inhibition of protein synthesis	No	A/E: gastritis, hyperphagia E: hyperglycemia, hypertension, mood swings, susceptibility to infections D: pancreatitis, osteopenia, Cushing's syndrome, avascular necrosis
Imatinib (Gleevec)	Metabolized in liver, excreted in kidney Inhibits the BCR-ABL tyrosine kinase by blocking the ATP binding site Hepatic metabolism, mainly by CYP3A4 Multiple drug interactions (grapefruit juice, warfarin)	No	E: rash, pruritis, fatigue, fever, diarrhea, nausea, vomiting E: pancytopenia, elevated LFTs, elevated bilirubin, peripheral edema
Rituximab	Anti-CD20 monoclonal antibody Causes lysis of pre-B and mature B lymphocytes by activating complement cascade and inducing apoptosis	No	A: infusion-related reactions: fever, chills, hypotension, headache, nausea, vomiting, bronchospasm, cytokine release syndrome (rare) A: allergic hypersensitivity/anaphylaxis reactions E: infection

NOTE: Toxicities: A = acute (time of infusion—minutes to days), E = early (days to weeks), D = delayed (during course of therapy—weeks to months), L = late (months to years posttreatment) N/V = nausea and vomiting

Interactions Between Methotrexate and Selected Commonly Used Drugs

Recommendations are based on literature where available and/or the characteristics (e.g., extent of protein binding, renal clearance including tubular secretion) of the potentially interacting drug. Decisions made for individual patients should take into consideration the clinical situation of the patient (e.g., induction versus consolidation therapy, renal and hepatic function), the methotrexate dose to be administered (low versus high) and the availability of alternative therapies.

Table 18-6   Interactions between methotrexate
and selected commonly used drugs.

Drug	Effect on Methotrexate Dose Intensity	Recommendation
Acyclovir	Likely ↑	Avoid
Amphotericin	Likely no direct effect	Consider another antifungal agent due to possible decreased renal function
Amoxicillin	↑	Avoid
Ampicillin	↑	Avoid
Cefaclor	Likely ↑	Avoid
Cefazolin	Likely ↑	Avoid
Cefotaxime	Likely ↑	Avoid
Ceftazidime	Likely none to minimal	OK
Ceftriaxone	Likely none	OK
Cefuroxime	Likely ↑	Avoid
Cephalexin	Likely ↑	Avoid
Ciprofloxacin	↑	Avoid
Clarithromycin	Likely none	Use cautiously
Clindamycin	Likely none	OK
Cloxacillin	Likely ↑	Avoid
Cotrimoxazole	↑	Avoid
Dapsone	Likely none to minimal	Use cautiously
Erythromycin	Likely none	OK
Fluconazole	Likely none	OK
Gentamicin	Likely none	OK
Meropenem	Likely ↑	Avoid
Metronidazole	Likely none	OK
Omeprazole	↑	Avoid
Oseltamivir	Likely ↑	Avoid
Pantoprazole	↑	Avoid
Penicillin g/v	Likely ↑	Avoid
Pentamidine	Likely none	OK
Piperacillin	Likely ↑	Avoid
Vancomycin	Likely none	OK

References

Adamson PC, Balis FM, Berg S, Blaney SM. General principles of chemotherapy. In: Pizzo PA, Poplack DG, ed. *Principles and Practice of Pediatric Oncology*. 5th ed. Philadelphia, PA: Lippincott Williams & Wilkins; 2006:294.

BC Cancer Agency. *Cancer Drug Manual*. http://www.bccancer.bc.ca/HPI/DrugDatabase/DrugIndexPro/default.htm. Accessed July 30, 2008.

Dalle JH, Auvrignon A, Vassal G, Leverger G. Interaction between methotrexate and ciprofloxacin. *J Pediatr Hematol Oncol*. 2002;24(4):321–322.

Joerger M, Huitema ADR, van den Bongard HJGD, et al. Determinants of the elimination of methotrexate and 7-hydroxy-methotrexate following high-dose infusional therapy to cancer patients. *Brit J Clin Pharmacol*. 2005;62:71–80.

Reid T, Yuen A, Catolico M, Carlson RW. Impact of omeprazole on the plasma clearance of methotrexate. *Cancer Chemother Pharmacol*. 1993;33:82–84.

Yamamoto K, Sawada Y, Matsushita Y, et al. Delayed elimination of methotrexate associated with piperacillin administration. *Ann Pharmacother*. 1997;31:1261–1262.

Zarychanski R, Wlodarczyk K, Ariano R, Bow E. Pharmacokinetic interaction between methotrexate and piperacillin/tazobactam resulting in prolonged toxic concentrations of methotrexate. *J Antimicrob Chemother*. 2006;58:228–230.

chapter 19

Guidelines For Drug Usage in Pediatric Oncology

Oussama Abla

Outline

- Drug Dosage Guidelines
- Blocked Central Venous Lines

Drug Dosage Guidelines

*Formulations for extemporaneously prepared products designated as 'SICKKIDS' may be available on the Compounding Service site at www.sickkids.ca/pharmacy.

Table 19-1 Drug dosage guidelines for children (please consult other handbooks for current neonatal drug dosing guidelines).

Supplied*	Dose
Acetaminophen Drops: 80 mg/mL Suspension: 80 mg/mL Tablets: 325 + 500 mg Chewtabs: 80 mg Suppositories: 120, 325 + 650 mg Suppository SICKKIDS: 60 mg	Analgesic: 15 mg/kg/dose PO q4–6h PRN Antipyretic: 10–15 mg/kg/dose PO q4–6h PRN
Acyclovir Suspension: 40 mg/mL Tablets: 200, 400, 800 mg Injection SICKKIDS: 6 mg/mL	**Dose on ideal body weight:** *Herpes simplex* encephalitis: 1 month–12 yrs: 60 mg/kg/day IV ÷ q8h × 14–21 days >12 yrs: 30 mg/kg/day IV ÷ q8h × 14–21 days Other *Herpes simplex,* including gingival stomatitis: Treatment: 15–30 mg/kg/day IV ÷ q8h Genital Herpes and other recurrent HSV infections: 200 mg PO QID Prophylaxis in immunocompromised hosts (other than HIV positive patients): 50 mg/kg/day PO ÷ QID Varicella or Zoster in immunocompromised hosts: <1 yr: 30 mg/kg/day IV ÷ q8h ≥1yr: 1500 mg/m²/day IV ÷ q8h; PO dosing (following IV therapy): 80 mg/kg/day PO ÷ QID
Allopurinol Suspension SICKKIDS: 20 mg/mL Tablets: 100 mg	200–300 mg/m²/day PO ÷ BID-QID 12 mg/kg/day PO ÷ BID-QID
Alteplase (Tissue plasminogen activator, tPA) Injection: 2 + 50 mg/vial	See Guidelines for Blocked Central Venous Lines page 362 Loculated Pleural Effusion via chest tube: Usual dose: 4 mg in 8 mL NaCl 0.9%; 2 mg in 4 mL NaCl 0.9% may be used in neonates and infants.

Dose Limit	Comments
75 mg/kg/day or 4 g/day if > 12 years old, whichever is less	Do not use acetaminophen for analgesia in neutropenic patients.
1 g/day PO	Maintain optimal hydration (1½ times maintenance) and urine output of at least 1 mL/kg/hr. Monitor accurate input/output and renal function. Minimize use of concurrent nephrotoxic agents whenever possible. May be given PO with food. Dose interval adjustment in renal impairment: Moderate (GFR 25–50 mL/min/1.73 m^2): q12h; Severe (GFR 10–25 mL/min/1.73 m^2): q24h. GFR <10 mL/min/1.73 m^2: 50% of dose q24h–48h. Haemodialysis: 50% of dose q24h (give after dialysis)
800 mg/day	Maintain fluid intake. Dose adjustment in renal impairment: Moderate: 50%; severe: 25–30%
	For chest tube administration, flush with 20–50 mL NaCl 0.9% Dose may be repeated after 1 hour.

(continued)

Table 19-1 (continued).

Supplied*	Dose
Aluminum Hydroxide & **Aluminum & Magnesium** **Hydroxides** Aluminum Hydroxide: Suspension: 64 mg/mL Chewtabs: 600 mg Aluminum + Magnesium Hydroxides: Magnesium Hydroxide 60 mg/mL Aluminium Hydroxide 99 mg/mL	Infant: 2.5–5 mL PO q1–2h Child: 5–15 mL PO pc & qhs Adult: 15–45 mL PO pc & qhs
Amikacin Injection: 250 mg/mL Injection SICKKIDS: 10 mg/mL	Patients with fever and neutropenia: Initial dose: 20–30 mg/kg/dose IV q24h
Amlodipine Suspension SICKKIDS: 1 mg/mL Tablet: 5 mg	Initial: 0.1–0.2 mg/kg/day PO as a single daily dose Maintenance: 0.1–0.4 mg/kg/day PO as a single daily dose
Amphotericin B Injection SICKKIDS: 0.1 mg/mL Ampho B Lipid Complex (Abelcet®) Ampho B Liposomal (Ambisome®)	Conventional amphotericin: 1–1.5 mg/kg/day IV once daily Empiric treatment: Ambisome®: 3 mg/kg/day IV once daily Treatment of suspected/actual infection: Abelcet®: 5 mg/kg/day IV once daily
Atovaquone	1–3 months and >2 yrs: 30 mg/kg/day PO as a single daily dose 4–24 months: 45 mg/kg/day PO as a single dose
Bisacodyl Tablet: 5 mg Suppositories: 5 + 10 mg	0.3 mg/kg/dose PO 6–12 hrs before desired effect. ≤6 yrs: 5–10 mg suppository PR 15–60 minutes before desired effect >6 yrs: 10 mg suppository PR 15–60 minutes before desired effect

Dose Limit	Comments
	After meals or pc (post cidum).
No dose limit.	Avoid in patients with significant pre-exisiting hearing loss or renal impairment (GFR <60 mL/min/1.73 m^2). Consider ciprofloxacin as substitute.
	Individualize doses based on serum concentrations obtained 3 & 6 hours after dose.
15 mg/day	Reduce initial dose in patients with hepatic impairment and titrate to effect. Due to the long half life of the drug, dosage adjustments should not be made more frequently than q3–5 days. Give at bedtime for cyclosporine-induced hypertension.
Conventional amphotericin: 70 mg/day or 1.5 mg/kg/dose whichever is less	Monitor serum potassium. Consider premedication with acetaminophen, meperidine, and diphenhydramine. Give NaCl 0.9% IV load 10 mL/kg before each amphotericin dose as tolerated.
1500 mg /dose	Give with food to ensure adequate absorption.
15 mg	Do not divide or chew tablets. Do not administer PO with dairy products or antacid.
	Do not administer suppositories pr to neutropenic patients.

(continued)

Table 19-1 (continued).

Supplied*	Dose
Calcium Solution: Calcium Glucoheptonate & Calcium Gluconate Suspension: SICKKIDS: Calcium Carbonate Tablets: Calcium Carbonate Injection: Calcium Chloride Calcium Gluconate	Calcium deficiency or initial dose for phosphate binding: Infants: 125 mg elemental calcium/dose PO TID cc (3.1 mmol elemental calcium/dose PO TID cc) Children: 250 mg elemental calcium/dose PO TID cc (6.25 mmol elemental calcium/dose PO TID cc) Hypocalcemia: 0.1–0.2 mmol elemental calcium/kg/hr IV Adjust IV rate q4h according to serum calcium concentration
Caspofungin Injection SICKKIDS: 7 mg/mL Injection: 50 + 70 mg/vial	Empiric therapy: Loading dose: 70 mg/m^2/dose IV q24h × 1 Maintenance dose: 50 mg/m^2/day IV as a single daily dose
Ceftazidime Injection: 1, 2 and 6 g/vials Injection SICKKIDS: 250 mg/mL	Mild to moderate infections: 100 mg/kg/day IV/IM ÷ q8h Severe infections: 125–150 mg/kg/day IV ÷ q8h
Cefuroxime Injection: 750 + 1500 mg/vials Injection SICKKIDS: 100 mg/mL	75–150 mg/kg/day IV/IM ÷ q8h
Ciprofloxacin Injection: 2 mg/mL Tablet: 250, 500 + 750 mg Suspension: 100 mg/mL	Patients with fever and neutropenia: 20 mg/kg/day IV ÷ q12h
Clindamycin Base: Injection SICKKIDS: 30 mg/mL Injection: 900 mg/vial	Piperacillin-allergic patients with fever and neutropenia: 30 mg/kg/day IV ÷ q8h

Dose Limit	Comments
	Titrate dose according to serum PO_4 or to corrected serum Ca. Avoid extravasation. A central venous line is preferred.
70 mg/dose	Reduce dose in hepatic impairment.
3 g/day	Dose interval adjustment in renal impairment:
6 g/day	Mild: q12h; Moderate: q24h; Severe: q48h
6 g/day	Not to be used for the treatment of meningitis. Dose interval adjustment in renal impairment: Moderate: q12h; severe: q24h.
800 mg/day IV	Dose interval adjustment in renal impairment: Moderate-severe: q18–24h May decrease clearance of warfarin, tacrolimus, cyclosporine, other drugs. Use with caution in patients with seizure disorders. Monitor for arthralgias, tendinitis. Maintain adequate fluid intake to prevent crystalluria.
600 mg/dose IV	In febrile neutropenia, consider stopping after 48hrs if cultures are negative.

(continued)

Table 19-1 (continued).

Supplied*	Dose
Cloxacillin Suspension: 25 mg/mL Capsules: 250 + 500 mg Injection: 0.5 + 2 g/vial Injection SICKKIDS: 100 mg/mL	Mild to moderate infections: 50–100 mg/kg/day PO/IV ÷ q6h Severe infections: 150–200 mg/kg/day IV/IM ÷ q6h
Codeine Syrup: 5 mg/mL Tablets: 15, 30 + 60 mg Injection: 30 mg/1 mL	Antitussive: 0.8–1.2 mg/kg/day PO ÷ q4–6h Analgesia dose: see chapter 13

Cotrimoxazole
Suspension:
trimethoprim 8 mg/mL +
  sulfamethoxazole 40 mg/mL
Pediatric Tablets:
trimethoprim 20 mg +
  sulfamethoxazole 100 mg
Adult Tablets:
trimethoprim 80 mg +
  sultamethoxazole 400 mg
Injection:
trimethoprim 16 mg/mL +
  sulfamethoxazole 80 mg/mL
	Bacterial infection:
	Treatment:
	8–12 mg trimethoprim/kg/day
	  PO/IV ÷ q12h
	(Includes 25–60 mg/kg/day
	  sulfamethoxazole)
	Prophylaxis:
	Urinary tract infection:
	2–5 mg trimethoprim/kg/day PO
	  once daily
	Asplenia and <6 months of age:
	5 mg trimethoprim/kg/day PO
	  once daily
	Pneumocystis jirovecii (carinii):
	Treatment:
	20 mg trimethoprim/kg/day IV/PO
	  ÷ q6h (includes 100 mg/kg/day
	  sulfamethoxazole)
	Prophylaxis:
	150 mg trimethoprim/m^2/day (5
	  mg TMP/kg/day) PO on 3 consec-
	  utive days of the week as a single
	  daily dose.

Dapsone
Tablet: 100 mg
Suspension: SICKKIDS: 2 mg/mL
	Pneumocystis jirovecii (carinii) Pro-
	  phylaxis in children >1 month:
	2 mg/kg/day PO once daily.
	OR
	4 mg/kg/day PO as a single dose
	  once weekly.

Dose Limit	Comments
4 g/day PO/IV	Give PO on an empty stomach (1 hr ac or 2 hrs pc).
12 g/day IV	
Antitussive: 20 mg/dose	Close clinical monitoring for dose-related toxicity recommended Maximum dose should not be given for >24 hrs.
320 mg TMP/day	Maintain fluid intake. May be given PO with food. Daily PO dose can be divided BID if once daily dose is not tolerated.
(160 mg TMP/dose) *Pneumocystis jirovecii (carinii)* prophylaxis: 320 mg TMP/day for 3×/weekly regimen	Dose interval adjustment in renal impairment: Moderate: q18h; Severe: q24h. Use with caution in patients with G-6–PD deficiency. Close clinical monitoring for dose-related toxicity recommended. Will decrease clearance of high dose methotrexate. Hold cotrimoxazole 48 hrs prior to high dose methotrexate, resume once methotrexate has cleared.
Daily dose: 100 mg/day Weekly dose: 200 mg/day	Close clinical monitoring for dose-related toxicity recommended. Monitor for methemoglobinemia and hemolysis. Use with caution in patients with G-6–PD deficiency or hypersensitivity to sulfonamnides. May cause photosensitivity. Do not administer with antacids.

(continued)

Table 19-1   (continued).

Supplied*	Dose
Desmopressin Intra-Nasal Solution: 0.25 mg/2.5 mL Intra-Nasal Spray: 2.5 mg/5 mL (10 microgram/spray) 2.5 mL Injection: 4 +15 microgram/1 mL Tablet: 100 + 200 microgram	Diabetes insipidus: Nasal: 5–20 microgram/day intranasally once daily or ÷ BID Oral: 100–1200 microgram/day PO ÷ BID-TID Coagulopathy (e.g., von Willebrand disease): 0.3 microgram/kg/dose IV/SC. May repeat after >12 hours if necessary.
Dexamethasone Suspension SICKKIDS: 1 mg/mL Tablets: 0.5 + 4 mg Injection: 20 mg/5 mL Injection: SICKKIDS: 0.4 mg/mL	Prevention of chemotherapy-induced nausea/vomiting: Very highly emetogenic regimens: 8 mg/m^2/dose PO/IV pre-chemo and q12h thereafter Highly emetogenic regimens: 4.5 mg/m^2/dose PO/IV pre-chemo and q12h thereafter Increased ICP: Initial: 0.2–0.4 mg/kg/IV Subsequent dose: 0.3 mg/kg/day IV/IM ÷ q6h
Dimenhydrinate Liquid: 3 mg/mL Tablets: 15 + 50 mg Suppositories: 25 + 50 mg Injection: 50 mg/1 mL	5 mg/kg/day PO/IV/IM/pr ÷ q6h
Diphenydramine Elixir: 2.5 mg/mL Tablet: 25 mg Capsule: 50 mg Injection: 50 mg/1 mL	Antihistamine: 5 mg/kg/day PO/IV/IM ÷ q6h Anaphylaxis: 1–2 mg/kg/dose IV

Dose Limit	Comments
Coagulopathy: 20 microgram/dose	Consider oral route for patients with diabetes insipidus who are unable to tolerate intranasal administration. Start with low dose and titrate to effect. Risk of severe hyponatremia. Restrict fluid intake and monitor fluid balance closely. Monitor serum electrolytes at baseline and repeat prior to each consecutive dose. No hypotonic fluids should be given intravenously. If serum Na+ <135 mmol/L, do not administer and contact prescriber for further directions. Due to risk of hyponatremia/seizures, use in children <3 yrs is generally contraindicated.
20 mg/dose Initial dose: 10 mg	Use of dexamethasone may be contraindicated if the antineoplastic protocol prohibits its use as an antiemetic or in patients receiving treatment for brain tumors. This contraindication may be reevaluated based on patient response. To discontinue inpatients receiving therapy for ≥10 days, reduce dose by 50% q48h until 0.3 ± 0.1 mg/m²/day achieved. Then reduce dose by 50% q10–14 days.
300 mg/day	Do not administer suppositories pr to neutropenic patients.
300 mg/day 50 mg/dose	

(continued)

Table 19-1 (continued).

Supplied*	Dose
Docusate Sodium Liquid: 4 mg/mL Capsule: 100 mg	5 mg/kg/day PO ÷ q6–8h or as a single daily dose
Domperidone Tablet: 10 mg Suspension: SICKKIDS: 1 mg/mL	1.2–2.4 mg/kg/day PO ÷ TID-QID Give 15–30 min ac + qhs
Filgrastim (G-CSF) Injection: 300 microgram/1 mL	5 micrograms/kg/day SC/IV as a single dose. If response is marginal after a cycle of chemo increase dose to: 10 micrograms/kg/day SC/IV as a single daily dose after next and subsequent cycles.
Fluconazole Suspension: 10 mg/mL Tablets: 50 + 100 mg Injection: 2 mg/mL	3–12 mg/kg/day PO/IV as a single dose Oropharyngeal candidasis: 3 mg/kg/day PO as a single daily dose Esophageal candidiasis: 3–6 mg/kg/day PO as a single daily dose Prophylaxis: AML: 5 mg/kg/day PO/IV as a single daily dose
Furosemide Liquid: 10 mg/mL Tablets: 20 + 40 mg Injection: 20 mg/2 mL, 250 mg/25 mL	1–2 mg/kg/day PO. May increase by 1–2 mg/kg/dose PO q6–8h PRN 0.5–2 mg/kg/dose IV/IM q6–12h

Dose Limit	Comments
Usual adult dose: 100–200 mg/day	Dilute liquid in milk or juice. Due to delayed onset of action, not recommended for PRN use.
80 mg/day Usual adult dose: 10 mg TID-QID	Dose adjustment in renal impairment as follows: extend interval to once or twice daily: consider dose reduction in more severe impairment. Use caution in patients with hepatic impairment.
10 micrograms/kg/day	Usual Discontinuation Endpoints: Antineoplastic therapy: ANC $\geq 1.5 \times 10^9$ on 2 consecutive days. Fever and Neutropenia: ANC $\geq 1 \times 10^9$ on 2 consecutive days, patient clinically improved, focus resolved & cultures negative.
400 mg/day	Use with caution in patients with liver impairment.
200 mg/day PO	Dose interval adjustment in renal impairment: Moderate: q48h; severe: q72h.
400 mg/day	OR adjust dose (not interval): moderate: 50%, severe: 25%. Hemodialysis: dose after each dialysis.
400 mg/day	Monitor carefully in patients also taking warfarin. May decrease clearance of tacrolimus, sirolimus cyclosporine, phenytoin and other medications.
PO: 6 mg/kg/dose or 80 mg/dose IV: 80 mg/kg/dose	

(continued)

Table 19-1 (continued).

Supplied*	Dose
Gabapentin Capsule: 100, 300 + 400 mg Suspension SICKKIDS: 100 mg/mL	Initial dose: 20–30 mg/kg/day PO ÷ TID Increase dose gradually over 3–7 days. Maintenance dose: 20–50 mg/kg/day PO ÷ TID Adolescents and adults: initial dose: 300 mg PO once on Day 1, 300 mg PO BID on Day 2, 300 mg PO TID on Day 3. Maintenance dose: 900–1800 mg/day PO ÷ TID
Ganciclovir Injection: SICKKIDS: 100 mg/mL	CMV infection: Treatment: 10 mg/kg/day IV ÷ q12h
Gentamicin Injection: 10 + 40 mg/mL	Patients with fever and neutropenia: Age Initial dose 1 mo–<9 yr 10 mg/kg/dose IV q24h 9–<12 yrs 8 mg/kg/dose IV q24h ≥12 yrs 6 mg/kg/dose IV q24h
Granisetron Injection: 1 mg/mL	Prevention of chemotherapy-induced nausea/vomiting: 20 microgram/kg/dose IV pre-chemo & q12h
Hydralazine Solution: SICKKIDS: 1 mg/mL, Tablets: 10–25, 50 mg Injection: 20 mg/1 mL	Initial dose: 0.15–0.8 mg/kg/dose IV q4–6h or 1.5 microgram/kg/min IV Maintenance dose: 0.75–7 mg/kg/day PO ÷ q6h

Dose Limit	Comments
3600 mg/day 2400 mg/day (long term)	Dose adjustment in renal impairment: mild: 50%; moderate: 25%; severe: 12.5%
	Consult product monograph for dose and interval adjustment in patients with impaired renal function.
No dose limit.	Avoid in patients with significant pre-existing hearing loss or renal impairment (GFR <60 mL/min/ 1.73 m^2). Consider ciprofloxacin as substitute. Individualize doses based on serum concentrations obtained 3 & 6 hours after dose.
	Use with caution in hepatic impairment.
20 mg/dose IV 7 mg/kg/day PO or 200 mg/day PO whichever is less.	Dose interval adjustment in renal impairment: Mild-moderate: q8h; severe: q8–24h Associated with development of drug induced lupus.

(continued)

Table 19-1 (continued).

Supplied*	Dose
Hydromorphone Injection: 2 mg/mL, 10 mg/mL Syrup 1 mg/mL	Intermittent IV: 15–20 microgram/kg/dose IV q2–4h Continuous infusion: 4–6 microgram/kg/hr IV Children ≤50 kg: 0.04–0.08 mg/kg/dose PO q3–4h PRN Children >50 kg: 2–4 mg/dose PO q3–4h PRN Patients with prior opiate exposure may tolerate higher doses
Hydroxyzine Syrup: 2 mg/mL Capsules: 10 + 25 mg	2 mg/kg/day PO ÷ TID or QID
Labetalol Injection: 100 mg/20 mL	Hypertension: 1 mg/kg/hour by continuous IV infusion. Acute hypertension: 1–3 mg/kg IV
Lactulose Syrup: 667 mg/mL	Constipation: Initial dose: 5–10 mL/day PO once daily Double daily dose until improvement
Lansoprazole Capsule: 15 + 30 mg Tablet, Oral Disintegrating (ODT): 15 + 30 mg	<10 kg: 7.5 mg PO once daily 10–30 kg: 15 mg PO once daily ≥30 kg: 30 mg PO once daily
Linezolid Injection: 600 mg/300 mL Tablet: 600 mg	Complicated infections, including Vancomycin-resistant *Enterococcus faecium* (VREF): <12 yrs: 30 mg/kg/day IV/PO ÷ q8h ≥12 yrs: 1200 mg/day IV/PO ÷ q12h
Loperamide Solution: 0.2 mg/mL Tablet: 2 mg	Acute diarrhea (initial dose in first 24 hrs): 2–5 yrs: 1 mg/dose PO TID 6–8 yrs: 2 mg/dose PO BID >8–12 yrs 2 mg/dose PO TID

Dose Limit	Comments
2–4 mg/dose PO (up to 8 mg/dose PO has been used)	Administer PO with or after food to decrease GI upset. If oral liquid spills on skin, remove contaminated clothing and rinse area with cool water.
400 mg/day	
3 mg/kg/hour	Reduce dose in liver impairment.
<1 yr: 2.5 mL PO QID Usual adult dose: 15–30 mL/day	
1.6 mg/kg/day or 30 mg/day, whichever is less	Administer prior to food. For oral use give capsules whole whenever possible.
600 mg/dose 1200 mg/dose	Usual duration is 10–14 days. For VREF, treatment duration is 14–28 days. Rare reports of serotonin syndrome when co-administered with SSRIs, TCAs, meperidine & other medications. Review carefully for potential drug interactions. Monitor CBC q weekly, and visual function if used for >3 mos.
	After initial dosing, 0.1 mg/kg after each loose stool, not exceeding initial dosage.

(continued)

Table 19-1 (continued).

Supplied*	Dose
Lorazepam Sublingual tablets: 0.5, 1, 2 mg Injection: 4 mg/1 mL	Treatment of breakthrough chemotherapy-induced nausea and vomiting: 0.025–0.05 mg/kg/dose IV/PO/SL q6h PRN
Meperidine Solution: SICKKIDS: 10 mg/mL Injection: 50 + 100 mg/1 mL	Prevention or treatment of amphotericin–induced rigors: 1–1.5 mg/kg/dose IV q3–4h PRN
Meropenem Injection: Supplied by pharmacy as 20 mg/mL ready to administrer solution.	Patients with fever and neutropenia: 60 mg/kg/day IV ÷ q8h Meningitis: 120 mg/kg/day IV ÷ q8h 6 g/day
Metoclopramide Liquid: 1 mg/mL Tablets: 5, 10 mg Injection: 10 mg/2 mL, 50 mg/10 mL	Gastro-esophageal reflux: 0.4–0.8 mg/kg/day PO/IM/IV ÷ QID Prevention or treatment of chemotherapy-induced nausea and vomiting: 1.5–2 mg/kg/dose IV pre-chemo and q2–4h Prevention of delayed chemotherapy-induced nausea and vomiting. 0.1–0.2 mg/kg/dose PO/IV q6h
Metronidazole Susp SICKKIDS: 15 mg/mL Tablet: 250 mg Injection: 500 mg/100 mL Injection: SICKKIDS: 5 mg/mL	Anaerobes: 15–30 mg/kg/day PO ÷ TID 30 mg/kg/day IV ÷ q6–8h *C difficile*: 35–50 mg/kg/day IV/PO ÷ q6h/QID
Mineral Oil (Heavy) Liquid	1 mL/kg/dose PO qhs

Dose Limit	Comments
4 mg/dose; 8 mg/12 hr or 0.1 mg/ kg/12 hrs whichever is less	Reduce dose in liver impairment. May give SL tablets PO For sublingual/buccal administration, dry saliva in region to ensure tablet dissolves and is absorbed in mucous membrane.
2 mg/kg dose or 100 mg/dose (whichever is less)	Avoid use in severe renal impairment. May cause constipation, respiratory or CNS depression. Dose is cumulative. Metabolite may cause seizures. Skin reactions and itching often respond to antihistamines and usually do not imply allergy.
6 g/day 3 g/day	Dose and interval adjustments in renal impairment: Mild: give standard dose q12h; moderate, give 50% dose q12h; severe: give 50% dose q24h. Dose after dialysis.
GER adult dose: 10–15 mg QID Antiemetic therapy: 10 mg/kg/day	May alter absorption of other drugs. When used as antiemetic, concomitant diphenhydramine is recommended.
2 g/day PO 4 g/day IV	Dose adjustment in renal impairment: Severe: 50% Hemodialysis: Dose after dialysis. Give PO with food or milk. Avoid alcohol. Suspension is chocolate-cherry flavoured but very bitter tasting. Trichomonas vaginalis: Partner must be treated.
Usual adult dose: 15–45 mL PO as a single dose	Avoid in children <1 yr.

(continued)

Table 19-1 (continued).

Supplied*	Dose

Morphine
Syrup: 1 mg/mL
Tablets: 5, 10 mg
Tablets. Sustained Release:
15, 30, 60, 100 mg
Capsules, Sustained Release
10, 15, 30 mg
Suppository: 5 mg
Injection: 2 mg/mL, 10 mg/mL, 15
  mg/mL, 50 mg/mL
Injection epidural: 5 mg/10 mL
	Analgesia:
	Intermittent dosing:
	0.2–0.4 mg/kg/dose PO/pr q4h or
	  0.05–0.1 mg/kg/dose IV/SC q2–
	  4h
	Continuous infusion:
	0.1–0.2 mg/kg IV loading dose
	0.01–0.04 mg/kg/hr IV/SC infusion
	0.02–0.05 mg/kg/dose IV/SC q4h
	  PRN for breakthrough pain
	Increase infusion rate q8h PRN in
	  increments ≤25% of previous
	  infusion rate.

Nabilone
Capsule: 0.5 + 1 mg
	Prevention of chemotherapy-
	  induced nausea and vomiting:
	<18 kg: 0.5 mg PO pre-chemo &
	  q12h
	18–30 kg: 1 mg PO pre-chemo &
	  q12h
	>30 kg: 1 mg PO pre-chemo &
	  q8–12h

Nadolol Suspension: SICKKIDS: 10 mg/mL Tablets: 40 + 80 mg	Hypertension: 1 mg/kg/day PO once daily or ÷ BID Increase dose by 1 mg/kg/day q3– 4 days PRN

Nifedipine
Capsules: 5 + 10 mg
	Acute management of hyperten-
	  sion: 0.25–0.5 mg/kg/dose PO
	  q4h PRN (minimum 1.25 mg/
	  dose)

Omeprazole
Delayed release tablet: 10 + 20 mg
Suspension SICKKIDS: 2 mg/mL
	Erosive esophagitis:
	1 month–2 yrs:
	1–3 mg/kg/day PO once daily or ÷
	  BID
	>2 yrs:
	0.7–2.5 mg/kg/day PO once daily
	  or ÷ BID

Dose Limit	Comments
IV/SC: 15 mg/dose No dose limit for palliative care.	Dosage adjustment in renal impairment: moderate: 75%; severe: 50%. Reduce dose in hepatic impairment. IM route should not be used for analgesia. Capsules may be opened and contents sprinkled on soft food. Pellets should not be chewed. Continuous IV/SC infusion is preferred to intermittent dosing for management of prolonged pain requiring frequent or high dose morphine administration. Dose may be safely titrated upwards. Do not adjust maintenance infusion dose until current dose has been running for at least 8 hrs. Reduce dose in hepatic impairment.
4 mg/kg/day or 320 mg/day whichever is less	Dose adjustment in renal impairment: Moderate: 50% Severe: 25%
10 mg/dose 2 mg/kg/day	Do not use in neonates. For more rapid action, direct patient to bite and swallow capsule.
3.5 mg/kg/day or 80 mg/day, whichever is less.	Reduce dose in hepatic impairment. Avoid splitting or crushing tablets if at all possible. Suspension to be used for G-tube administration.

(continued)

Table 19-1 (continued).

Supplied*	Dose
Ondansetron Tablets: 4 + 8 mg Liquid: 0.8 mg/mL Injection: 4 mg/2 mL, 8 mg/4 mL Tablet, Oral Disintegrating (ODT): 4 + 8 mg	Prevention of chemotherapy-induced nausea and vomiting: Highly to very highly emetogenic antineoplastic regimen: 5 mg/m^2/dose IV/PO pre-chemo and q12h Moderate emetogenic regimen: 5 mg/m^2/dose IV/PO pre-chemo and q12h Low emetogenic regimen: 3 mg/m^2/dose IV/PO × 1 pre-chemo
Pantoprazole Injection: 40 mg/vial	Indications (GERD, acid suppression) requiring a proton pump inhibitor and the oral route is not feasible: 1–1.5 mg/kg/day IV once daily Upper Gastrointestinal (GI) Bleeding: 5–15 kg: 2 mg/kg/dose IV × 1 and then 0.2 mg/kg/hr IV >15–40 kg: 1.8 mg/kg/dose IV × 1 and then 0.18 mg/kg/hr IV >40 kg: 80 mg/dose IV × 1 and then 8 mg/hr IV
PEG (Polyethylene Glycol) 3350 NF Powder (PEGFlakes®)	4–8 kg: 4.25 g PO daily 9–16 kg: 8.5 g PO daily ≧17 kg: 17 PO daily
Pentamidine Isethionate Injection: 300 mg/vial	*Pneumocystis jirovecii* (carinii): Treatment: 4 mg/kg/day IV as a single daily dose for 14–21 days Prophylaxis: 4 mg/kg/dose IV q 2 weeks OR 300 mg/dose by inhalation q month.

Dose Limit	Comments
8 mg/dose	
40 mg/dose Maximum rate: 8 mg/hr 80 mg/dose Maximum infusion duration: 72 hours	For indications other than GI bleeding, gastric pH may be monitored as clinically necessary. For upper GI bleeding, gastric pH should be monitored to maintain pH >6.
17 g/day	Mix in approximately 120–240 mL of suitable beverage (water, juice or soda). Drink once dissolved. Onset of action: 2–4 days. Dose interval adjustment in renal impairment: Moderate: q24–36h; Severe: q48h Monitor for hypo/hyperglycemia, pancreatitis and rash. Give IV over 1 hour. Monitor for hypotension during infusion. Inhalation generally reserved for patients >5 yrs.

(continued)

Table 19-1 (continued).

Supplied*	Dose
Phytonadione (Vitamin K$_1$) Injection: 1 mg/0.5 mL, 10 mg/1 mL	Warfarin Antidote: No bleeding, future need for warfarin: 0.5–2 mg/dose PO No bleeding, no future need for warfarin OR significant bleeding, not life-threatening: 2–5 mg/dose PO or IV over 10–20 minutes. Significant bleeding, life-threatening: 5 mg/dose IV over 10–20 minutes
Piperacillin-Tazobactam (e.g. Tazocin®) Injection: 3.375 g (piperacillin 3 g + tazobactam 0.375 g) 4/5 g (piperacillin 3 g + tazobactam 0.5 g)	240 mg piperacillin/kg/day IV ÷ q8h
Prednisolone, Prednisone Prednisolone: Liquid: 1 mg base/mL Prednisone: Suspension: SICKKIDS: 5 mg/mL Tablets: 1, 5 + 50 mg	PCP Pneumonia: 1.6 mg/kg/day PO ÷ BID × 5 days, then 0.8 mg/kg/day as a single daily dose × 5 days, then 0.4 mg/kg/day as a single daily dose × 11 days
Ranitidine Solution: 15 mg/mL Tablets: 75, 150 mg Injection: 50 mg/2 mL	2–4 mg/kg/day IV ÷ q6–8h Peptic ulcer, gastro-esophageal reflux: Treatment: 5–10 mg/kg/day PO ÷ q12h × 8 weeks Maintenance: 2.5–5 mg/kg/day PO once daily ÷ BID
Rasburicase Injection: 1.5 mg/mL	0.2 mg/kg/dose IV over 30 minutes q24h. Evaluate serum urate concentration before giving subsequent doses.

Dose Limit	Comments
	Injection may be given by mouth, undiluted. Severe anaphylactoid rections have occurred with IV administration; give IV in emergency situations only.
100 mg piperacillin/kg/dose or 4 g piperacillin/dose, whichever is less	Dose and interval adjustment in renal impairment: Moderate: decrease dose by 39% + give q6h Severe: decrease dose by 30% + give q8h
40 mg PO BID × 5 days, then 40 mg PO daily × 5 days, then 20 mg PO daily × 11 days	For patients requiring oral liquid, which is very bitter-tasting, consider using prednisolone liquid (commercially available: Pediapred®, 1 mg base/mL). 1 mg prednisolone base = 1 mg prednisone
200 mg/day IV Max dose: 300 mg BID PO	Monitor gastric pH in patients requiring IV therapy. Dose adjustment in renal impairment: Moderate: 75%; Severe: 50%
	Contraindicated in G6PD deficiency. Dose according to ideal body weight in obese patients. Send blood samples for determination of urate concentration to the lab on ice for at least 96 hrs after rasburicase. Monitor for allergy. Do not give for longer than 7 days.

(continued)

Table 19-1 (continued).

Supplied*	Dose
Senna Syrup: 1.7 mg/mL Tablet: 8.6 mg	Syrup: 2–5 yrs: 3–5 mL/dose PO qhs 6–12 yrs: 5–10 mL/dose PO qhs Tablet: 6–12 yrs: 1–2 tablets/dose PO qhs
Sevelamer Tablet: 800 mg	Initial dose: 400 mg PO BID with meals. Titrate dose to serum phosphorus. Usual dose: 800–1600 mg PO TID with meals. Additional doses may be required with snacks.
Sodium Polystyrene Sulfonate (Kayexalate®) Powder Suspension: 250 mg/mL Enema: 30 g/120 mL	1 g/kg/dose PO q6h PRN 1 g/kg/dose PR q2–6h PRN
Tobramycin Injection: 10 mg/mL, 40 mg/mL, 80 mg/2 mL	Patients with fever and neutropenia: Age Initial dose 1 mo–<9 yr 10 mg/kg/dose IV/IM q24h 9–<12 yrs 8 mg/kg/dose IV/IM q24h ≥12 yrs 6 mg/kg/dose IV/IM q24h
Trimethoprim Suspension: SICKKIDS: 10 mg/mL Tablet: 100 mg	4–6 mg/kg/day PO ÷ q12h UTI prophylaxis: 2 mg/kg/day PO ÷ BID or as a single daily dose
Ursodiol Tablet: 250 mg Suspension: SICKKIDS: 60 mg/mL	10–20 mg/kg/day PO ÷ BID-TID

Dose Limit	Comments
Usual adult dose: 2–4 tablets PO qhs	
	Do not chew or split tablet. Separate administration from other PO medications whenever possible, giving them at least 1 hour before or 3 hours after sevelamer.
Usual adult oral dose: 15 g/dose	Exchange approximately 1 mmol/g of resin. Administer rectally in appropriate volume of tap water. D10W or equal parts tap water and 2% methylcellulose. Moisten resin with honey or jam for PO use.
No dose limit.	Avoid in patients with significant pre-existing hearing loss or renal impairment (GFR <60 mL/min/1.73 m^2). Consider ciprofloxacin as substitute. Individualize doses based on serum concentrations obtained 3 & 6 hours after dose.
Usual adult dose: 200 mg/day 100 mg/day	Dose interval adjustment in renal impairment: Moderate: q18h; severe: avoid May be given with food.
45 mg/kg/day	

(continued)

Table 19-1 (continued).

Supplied*	Dose
Vancomycin Capsule: 125 mg Liquid: SICKKIDS: 100 mg/mL Injection: SICKKIDS: 100 mg/mL Injection: 0.5, 1, 5 + 10 g/vial	Mild to moderate infections: 40 mg/kg/day IV ÷ q6h Severe infections: 40–60 mg/kg/ day IV ÷ q6h Unstable neutropenic patient with fever: 60 mg/kg/day IV ÷ q6h Meningitis: 60 mg/kg/day IV ÷ q6h *C. difficile* colitis: 50 mg/kg/day PO ÷ q6h
Voriconazole Injection: 200 mg/vial Tablets: 200 mg	**IV** Children: 2–11 yrs: 7 mg/kg/dose q12h Children: >12 yrs: Loading dose: 6 mg/kg/dose q12h for 2 doses on day 1 then: Maintenance dose: Invasive aspergillosis: 4 mg/kg/dose q12h Candidemia and other fungal infections: 3–4 mg/kg/dose q12h If patient cannot tolerate 4 mg/kg/ dose, reduce to 3 mg/kg/dose **Oral:** <40 kg: Invasive aspergillosis: Loading dose: 200 mg q12h × 2 doses Maintenance dose: 100 mg BID Candidemia and invasive candidiasis: Loading dose: 400 mg q12h × 2 doses Maintenance dose: 100 mg BID may increase to 150 mg/dose if needed ≥40 kg: Invasive aspergillosis: Loading dose: 400 mg q12h × 2 doses Maintenance: 200 mg BID Candidemia and invasive candidiasis: Loading dose: 400 mg q12h × 2 doses Maintenance dose: 200 mg BID may increase to 300 mg/dose if needed

Adapted with permission from Lau E(ed). 2008–2009 Drug Handbook and Formulary. Sick Kids; Toronto, 2008.

Dose Limit	Comments
2 g/day 4 g/day prior to TDM (drug levels) 4 g/day prior to TDM 4 g/day prior to TDM	Calculate doses according to effective body weight. Dose interval adjustment in renal failure as follows: mild: q8–12h, moderate: q18–48h; severe: q3–7 day. Individualize doses based on trough serum concentrations. In febrile neutropenia, consider stopping after 48 hrs if cultures are negative. Injection may be used for oral dosing. Reduce dose in hepatic impairment. Interacts with other medications including cyclosporine, tacrolimus, sirolimus, omprazole and anticonvulsants. Monitor carefully for potential drug interactions. Oral tablets: have improved absorption if given at least 1 hour before or 1 hour after a meal. Visual changes such as blurred vision, photophobia, changes in visual acuity and color have been reported in 30% of patients in clinical trials. Dose individualization based on steady state trough serum voriconazole concentrations is recommended in cases of invasive fungal infection.

Blocked Central Venous Lines

The following are guidelines for management of blocked central venous lines (CVLs). Modifications for individual circumstances may be necessary. Consult latest edition of *SickKids' Formulary* for most current policy. In general, consultation from the thrombosis service should be obtained.

Indications

- For CVLs that are blocked and will not infuse properly.
- For CVLs that require blood return as an essential function, such as hematology/oncology catheters, hemodialysis catheters.
- All patients with clinical symptoms such as head/neck swelling, respiratory distress, bluish color, collateral circulation should be evaluated by objective tests such as venography, ultrasound and ventilation perfusion lung scans, and CT scans, as appropriate.

Initial Management

Complete chest X-ray (CXR) to visualize CVL placement

Table 19-2   Initial Management of blocked CVL's.

	Chemical-Related Blockage	Blood-Related Blockage
Indications	Infusion running then sudden unexplained occlusion	Blood sampling Blood administration Blood back-up in infusion
Initial Action	1. Attempt to aspirate 2. Flush with 0.9% NaCl 3. Follow HCL guidelines 4. If no blood return, follow guidelines for alteplase. If unsuccessful clearing the CVL contact interventional radiology (IGT). 5. If able to flush line but no blood return, proceed to diagnostic workup if clinically indicated. 6. If unable to flush line, contact IGT.	1. Attempt to aspirate 2. Flush with 0.9% NaCl 3. Follow guidelines for alteplase. If unsuccessful clearing the CVL contact IGT. 4. If able to flush line, but unable to get blood return, proceed to diagnostic workup if clinically indicated. 5. If unable to flush line, contact IGT.

Table 19-3 Guidelines For Local Instillation.

Type of Catheter	Chemical Occlusion	Blood-Related Occlusion	
	Hydrochloric Acid (HCL) 0.1 M	Size of Patient	Alteplase (tPA)
Single lumen (e.g., CVL, PICC)	2 ml	>10 kg	1 mg/ml. Use amount required to fill volume of line to maximum 2 ml = 2 mg.
		≤10 kg	1 mg diluted to 2 ml 1 ml = 0.5 mg
Double lumen (CVL, PICC, percutaneous CVL)	2 ml per lumen	>10 kg	1 mg/ml. Use amount required to fill volume of line to maximum 2 ml = 2 mg per lumen. Treat one lumen at a time.
		≤ 10 kg	1 mg diluted to 2 ml per lumen. 1 ml = 0.5 mg
Subcutaneous ports	3 ml	>10 kg	2 mg diluted with NS to 3 ml. 1 ml = 0.65 mg.
		≤10 kg	1.5 mg diluted with NS to 3 ml. 1 ml = 0.5 mg.
Hemodialysis catheters small Quinton large Quinton	1 ml 1.5 ml	>10 kg	See guidelines for single lumen catheter.
For non-Nephrology patients use double lumen guidelines		≤10 kg	0.75 mg diluted to 1.5 ml

Note: After a minimum of 2 hours instillation of each drug, withdraw drug; if possible, flush the catheter with NS and attempt to aspirate blood. Two trials of alteplase (tPA) local instillation may be attempted within a 24-hour period.

Diagnostic Work-Up

Investigation of a blocked CVL is necessary if the line fails to function properly after two doses of tPA, or if it has blocked for a second time. In certain situations, detailed investigation may be warranted even outside of these guidelines.

1. Perform a lineogram to determine the following:
   a. Location of the CVL.
   b. Potential occlusion at the tip of the CVL.
   c. Presence of retrograde flow.
   d. Potential leak.
   e. Lineogram cannot rule out the presence of large vessel clot, therefore must proceed as follows:
2. Perform a venogram.
   a. If the venogram is normal and the CVL is not functioning, then local occlusion must be present.
   b. If the venogram is abnormal, proceed to treatment as outlined below.
3. If a venogram (the "gold standard" investigation) cannot be readily obtained, perform a Doppler ultrasound evaluation of the large vessels near and including the CVL. However, the sensitivity and specificity of this technique for detection of large vessel thrombus in the upper venous system (especially intrathoracic vessels) is poor (20%). Venography remains the recommended investigation. Doppler is more sensitive (80%) than venogram in diagnosing neck vessel thrombosis.
   a. If the Doppler ultrasound and lineogram are normal but there is still no blood return from the CVL,

consider using the CVL for instillation only. Venogram is strongly recommended to rule out large vessel clot. Echocardiogram should be considered to rule out intracardiac thrombosis.

b. If the Doppler ultrasound and/or lineogram are abnormal (i.e., obstruction of flow related to occlusion at the tip of the catheter or retrograde flow around the catheter), it is recommended to proceed to a venogram to rule out proximal clot.

Treatment

Consult interventional radiology and a pediatric thrombosis specialist.

- Extensive deep vein thrombosis:
  a. 30% of children with DVT have pulmonary embolism (PE) and are asymptomatic. In cases of suspected PE, perform a chest XR. If normal, perform a ventilation/perfusion (V/Q) scan. If abnormal, perform a spiral CT scan.
  b. The following are options for management:
    - Leave the CVL in place and attempt local or systemic thrombolytic therapy if there are no contraindications.
    - Remove the CVL: Consult thrombosis specialist and treat with anticoagulation for 3–5 days before removing CVL.

Index